How I Overcame
PSORIASIS

How I Overcame

PSORIASIS

Kent Trussell

SALLY MILNER PUBLISHING

Dedication

To my wife and children

First published in 2001 by
Sally Milner Publishing Pty Ltd
PO Box 2104
Bowral NSW 2576
AUSTRALIA

© Kent Trussell 2001

Design by Anna Warren, Warren Ventures Pty Ltd, Sydney

Chapter illustrations by Anna Warren, Warren Ventures Pty Ltd, Sydney

Diagrams by Jessica Trussell

Edited by Anne Savage

Printed in Australia

Cover detail: *Male Torso, 1998* by Miranda Lean, Bundanoon, NSW

National Library of Australia Cataloguing-in-Publication data:
Trussell, Kent. 1951 -
   How I overcame psoriasis.

   Bibliography.

   Includes index.
   ISBN 1 86351 283 7.

   1. Psoriasis - Popular works. 2. Psoriasis - Treatment - Popular works. 3. Skin.
   I. Title.(Series : Milner health series).

616.526

Contents

Figures

Acknowledgments

This book would not have been possible without the tireless assistance of my wife, Deborah White, who was instrumental in its inception and has been responsible for most of the new research.

Our daughter Jessica did the line drawings, and our son Oliver offered valued feedback and opinion.

Thank you also to my mother, Avon Simpson, and my brother Philip Simpson, for proofreading the manuscript and compiling the bibliography.

Gratitude is also extended to Jill Turland of the Australian Homeopathic Association and osteopath Andrew Hall for their contributions to the discourses on these modalities.

The title, 'How I Overcame Psoriasis', was first used for an article commissioned for the May/June 1984 edition of *Australian Wellbeing* magazine by its publisher/editor, Barbara McGregor.

Preface

For the many sufferers of this puzzling skin disease who are searching for just a clue to its origins and liberation from their uncomfortable and (for some) unsightly affliction, the answers, as I found with a little research, personal adaptation and perseverance, are relatively simple.

So I wrote in the Introduction to *Sor-i-a-sis* in 1981. This present book is also intended to inform fellow psoriatics, and anyone else who is interested, of my success in achieving self-healing and control of the disease psoriasis. I hope that it might also serve as a guide for those interested in pursuing self-help. Please note however, that the involvement of a professional practitioner is considered essential. The tenacity and variable nature of the condition can mean that what works well for one person does not necessarily work for another.

Sor-i-a-sis was a collection of thoughts and suggestions for sufferers of the skin disease psoriasis. Within six months in the year before its publication I had reversed an approximately 80 per cent body cover to obtain a totally clear skin. Formerly, I had suffered from psoriasis for at least eighteen years. I achieved this reversal largely on my own account, as a result of research and determination. I was an idealist then and proclaimed a sincere belief that diet, lifestyle and how we think about ourselves are at the core of all illnesses and therefore of positive healing.

Sor-i-a-sis was subtitled 'Heal Yourself'. I rather loosely interpreted *Sor-i-a-sis* as the composite of ills that inflict the earth, and that personal afflictions such as this disease are mere symptoms of an overriding malaise which urgently needed to be confronted and resolved. The only people who could achieve this, I believed, were the 'sufferers'—you and me and everyone else on this planet who is sufficiently awake to the need and the means to accomplish this.

Well, I am still idealistic and still hold this belief along with others that were expounded then. Therefore my ideas on self-healing remain pretty much as they did in 1981. I am still a psoriatic. However, I have never again been afflicted as severely as in 1980, and only have to contend with an occasional spot here or there, providing I 'practise what I preach'. While these 'little spots' have sometimes become many, I have remained triumphant over my affliction and know how to treat it.

I know that what is suggested in these pages might not be useful to everybody, particularly to those who are merely expecting someone to produce a rapid-fire cure. I think, however, that the book's usefulness will depend on one's desire or willingness to try something, whether it be new or timeless. Ultimately it becomes a question of the level of commitment to one's self. For those people who want the boots-and-all panacea, wait and see what research in bioengineering will unfold. The psoriatic may then have the opportunity to decide the morality or otherwise of contributing to commercial processes which are underscored by 'ownership' of a key to a means of altering human experience. Meanwhile, the physiological impairment that is inherent in our degenerative disease, if it is still not tackled, will merely manifest itself in other forms.

For now, I understand the impracticability for many people of maintaining the determined dietary and lifestyle program which, at least in my experience, is necessary to eradicate the disease. We can be rid of this rotten affliction if we are so determined. Naturally this requires wholehearted involvement. I accept, however, that not a lot of people are in the position to pursue 'perfection'—myself amongst them. Therefore my immediate, practical advice is to arrest the current condition, gain remission, and find a balance that suits individual needs and circumstances, so one can live comfortably and positively with this 'differentness'.

Psoriasis is one of those diseases that orthodox medicine regards as being incurable. Why should anything be incurable? Rather, I believe in the power of the mind, and that setting the mind to achieve something is one of the best forces we can employ. I have willed psoriasis from my body.

The power of the mind is one of a number of avowals which it is important to establish from the outset. Some others are:

- We determine the nature of our own reality.
- All existence is blessed.
- The point of power is now.

Ultimately, you decide every aspect of your life. There is no thing better or worse than you. No person, thing or 'god' is to blame for who and what you are, and there is no such thing as 'bad' or 'good'. And finally, if you want something, now is the time to set in motion the things which will achieve everything you want.

If any of these statements challenges your beliefs or offends you, maybe your life is affected by false realities and beliefs—conditioning that can make you ill. You have possibly also assigned your personal power to some other person or 'thing'.

What is your reaction to the statement, 'You decided to have psoriasis'? Could it be possible that you decided to have this disease because (a) you believe that you earned it or deserve it and (b) having this disease attracts sympathy and attention to you, responses which you don't believe you are worthy of without inflicting some sort of self-punishment?

Louise L. Hay describes psoriatics as individuals who fear being hurt and refuse to accept responsibility for their own feelings. By accepting psoriasis we are deadening the senses and our self. For several years before reading this, I had thought of the patches of psoriasis on my elbows and knees as being like blinkers on a horse and that possibly, therefore, I was blinkering myself to other realities, not willing to see truths and so on. Elsewhere I had come upon the notion that our elbows and knees are psychic windows to our past. In Ms Hay's theory, the elbow represents changing directions and accepting new experiences, while the knee represents pride and ego. Problems associated with the knee denote stubborn ego and pride, an inability to bend, inflexibility, and refusal to give in.

What are we to make of these ideas? Perhaps they should be set aside, for to labour them could merely whittle another rod with which to flail ourselves. The new approach we are going to take is along more positive pathways; if we are going to assume an active role in achieving freedom from the cloak of psoriasis, we have to start by feeling good about ourselves. This book strives to provide clear examples of these processes, and to sow the seeds of other realities which the reader might care to explore.

It is also the purpose of this work to invite the collaboration of orthodox practitioners who will think outside the square—to treat patients wholistically, and through this to accept the efficacy and scope of alternative approaches. Orthodox and non-orthodox treatments can work in symbiosis, as complementary modalities. This dis-ease can be overcome.

This book is nowhere near complete as an encyclopaedia of the available information. That is the work's nature, however—to be an information exchange that is ongoing and updated. It has been very interesting throughout the process of researching new material, to realise how much of what is relevant has been known and discussed for many years. Clear advice on the role of diet and lifestyle, knowledge of the probable role of intestinal permeability in many psoriatics' indisposition, and understanding of important psychological factors, have been available for decades. Why then are there still so many millions of us wondering what the hell we can do to alleviate our suffering? Why are we still paying mega-millions of our hard-earned cash to be told we can't do anything better than poison ourselves further with some questionable lotion or pill?

Let's do this thing ourselves. If you have something to add to the information provided here, please join The Information Exchange. Ultimately, if we are to be rid of psoriasis, we must accept the intrinsic need for change, and we are the best people to kick off the process. By taking these steps, may we also work some good for all.

Good health!

Kent Trussell
2001

To the reader

Control of psoriasis can be achieved by treating the skin's surface (to gain relief from discomfort and heal the imbalance present here), by examining dietary and metabolic individuality (because of the need to detoxify and manage the degenerative nature of the disease) and by adopting a determined attitude (by establishing a firm desire for, and expectation of, being healed, and understanding the role of emotions in the diseased state).

Without wishing to slip into oversimplification, much of the information provided in the early pages is deliberately basic 'text book' in its nature and style. Many readers will already appreciate the importance of diet and lifestyle in maintaining good health. Overall, the aim is to provide useful information for all psoriatics, and through this, inspire a desire to explore other ideas and methodologies.

Note: Australian English and imperial measurements have been used throughout this book.

Suggestions for using this book

Part I: What Have We Got, and What Can We Do About It? provides basic, straightforward details of the vital body functions and their relationship with psoriasis. This also serves as an introduction to Part III.

Part II: Diary of a Psoriatic, contains my personal case history as a psoriatic since the age of ten until the time of writing, at age 49.

Part III: Taking Control, elaborates on vital and additional factors introduced in Part I, outlines worthwhile treatments, and introduces complementary therapies and other useful concepts.

Part III is divided into major sections as they are pertinent to treatment of this disease—surface healing, diet and 'internal' factors, and the important roles of the mind and our relationship with intrinsic energies.

The tables in Appendix 1 contain much of the information discussed in the book in condensed form.

Appendix 2, Information Exchange provides selected extracts from the personal experiences of other psoriatics whose own insight into self-healing is offered. Readers are invited to participate in this ongoing process of research and information sharing.

Disclaimer

The information in this instruction book is presented in good faith. However, no warranty is given, nor results guaranteed, nor is freedom from any patent to be inferred. Since we have no control over the use of information contained in this book, the publisher and the author disclaim liability for untoward results.

PART I

What have we got, and what can we do about it?

1 What is psoriasis?

Some facts about psoriasis

PSORIASIS NEED NOT BE A COMPLICATED PHENOMENON

As a skin disorder, psoriasis is the surface symptom of an imbalance within the whole body system.

The 'whole body system' is an individual entity with skin, a highly intelligent physiological, biochemical and electrical machine, and a mind.

This system's homeostasis is dependent on nourishment and a stable psychological framework.

THE SKIN

The scaly surface is the visible result of an abnormally rapid regeneration of cells

- The dead skin must be removed to promote healing.
- There are some very pleasant ways to achieve this.
- In addition to the skin of the body trunk, arms, legs and scalp, psoriasis can affect the eyelashes, eyelids and eyebrows and in extreme cases erode the cornea, and appear as conjunctivitis.

Extraordinary losses of vitamins and minerals occur with the condition

- If unchecked, this can weaken bone structure.
- Weakened bone structure causes chronic damage.
- Vitamins and minerals can be restored.

THE INTERNAL BODY

Psoriasis is aggravated by numerous substances, including alcohol, animal protein, saturated fats, gluten, and processed and refined foods

- The way each body uses nutrients—its metabolism—shares many characteristics with other human bodies and yet each is unique.
- Diet is crucial.
- Maintaining proper nutrition is made increasingly difficult by the

insurgence of toxins into fresh food production and the results of food processing.

The body is a living, biochemical and electrical entity
- It is designed to heal itself.
- Sufficient information and knowledge is extant, to enable us to help the body achieve this.
- It is an individual responsibility to pursue this course of action.

THE MIND

The mind can control how the body 'is'
- Stress can aggravate and cause illness.
- I have the power to influence physiological, biochemical and neurological changes in my body.
- I can change my life if I decide to.

Psoriasis has hereditary links
- Genes are merely a part of the biochemical and electrical machine.
- The mind is infinitely more powerful.
- I have control over my past, present and future.

To understand and gain control of psoriasis is to treat the condition on the surface, internally and emotionally.

* * *

There are very many disorders that topically affect the skin. They include dermatitis, cysts, diseases of nails and hair, drug reactions, eczema, phototoxicity, pigmentation disorders, psoriasis, tumours, ulcers, vitiligo and warts. It is not the intention or purpose of this edition to investigate these except for the king and queen of them all, psoriasis.

There are several variations of this common, tenacious and idiosyncratic condition that has been known for millennia. Various estimates place the number of psoriatics worldwide at anywhere between 1 and 5 per cent of the total population. Approximately 40 per cent of sufferers have psoriasis on the scalp. We have very many compatriots in our search for relief and understanding. Millions of us are irritated, uncomfortable and anxious. We often don't like to be seen in public, our personal life can be non-existent, and we hurt.

Meanwhile, we are worth a fortune to our nations' economies. Total annual expenditure on psoriasis treatment in the USA exceeds $1.5 billion; our North American counterparts spent upwards of $800 each on their personal experience with the disease in 2000.[1]

Ours is a very versatile disorder: it is not essentially or exclusively dermatological and, unlike many other complaints, it nurtures interest from and provides support for numerous medical disciplines, amongst them endocrinology, pathophysiology and genetics; dietetics, paediatrics and orthopaedics; rheumatology, psychology and psychiatry; and ophthalmology and photobiology. Natural health—alternative medicine—is involved in psoriasis treatment to a very large degree.

Clinical description

In its topical manifestations untreated psoriasis forms a thick, crusty, silvery or whitish, dry, scaly layer of dead skin cells (plaques). The plaque is the result of highly accelerated skin cell growth and decay (excessive keratinocyte differentiation—the psoriatic's skin 'differentiates' about 1,000 times faster than everyone else's). Clinically speaking, the plaque which we peel and pick at is a collection of immature cells that have reached the skin's surface and, retaining their nuclei, are not perfectly keratinised (parakeratinised). They adhere to the surface rather than being cast off as they would be under the normal process of keratinisation, and become dry and porous.

In all forms of the disease, the redness or inflammation beneath the crusty layer is caused by the build-up of blood which is required to feed the rapidly dividing cells. The pinpoints of dilated capillaries are visible when the plaques are scratched away and, if excessively scratched, can be made to bleed and reveal an irritated, bloody dewiness.

Psoriasis can be very itchy, especially when the patches are spread over a wide area of skin, and in a hot, humid climate. However, even the tiniest nummular spot can be itchy.

Precipitating factors

The first onset of psoriasis in those who are predisposed to it can occur at any age, although it has been shown that the predominantly susceptible years correspond with the most active periods of life, and for both men and women are between the ages of 10 and 35. It can occur in infants and in early childhood; it can also appear for the first time in old age.

The condition is clinically regarded as an inborn peculiarity in which the skin symptomatically reacts. Most commonly there is a stimulating cause present within the body that produces symptoms by working through the blood supply, lymphatic system and/or the nervous system. Certain conditions and experiences can precipitate or aggravate psoriasis, either on their own or in combination, including:

- Infective conditions, e.g. abscesses or ulcers, influenza, quinsy, tonsillitis, upper respiratory tract infections
- Nervous shock or strain which results from or is precipitated by accidents, surgical operations, and environmental or domestic upsets
- Vaccination
- Some prescription drugs
- Hormonal activity, e.g. puberty, menopause
- Pregnancy
- Menstruation and premenstrual tension
- Ordinary dermatitis
- Irritant applications or clothing

An eruption can also arise as the result of an injury to the skin (called the Koebner phenomenon), which can occur either during an existing attack or introduce a new one. Not in any way is psoriasis contagious.

Susceptibility appears to follow racial lines, with Caucasians the greatest number of sufferers. It is rarely known amongst Native North and South Americans. African Americans and West Africans usually have little experience of it. East Africans on the other hand are susceptible.[2] It also occurs amongst Australian Aboriginal and Torres Strait Islanders. It has not been known amongst the Inuit and is not generally known amongst Asians.

Psoriasis often first appears as a rash or red patches covered with the characteristic dry scales (*nummular psoriasis*). Individual spots appear in a small, roughly circular shape, sometimes in a symmetrical formation on both sides of the body. If untreated the spots can expand and spread to join with other patches. The speed and severity with which this happens have a direct relationship with the individual's general state of health. As the spots expand, they can leave clear skin at the centre (*annular psoriasis*).

The skin areas most commonly affected are the knees and elbows, the lower back, ears and scalp. Untreated and even treated patches tend to grow larger before remission is obtained. Psoriasis should heal without scarring; however, darker pigmentation is sometimes apparent, and this can be influenced by the nature and quality of the topical applications used in treatment. Spontaneous remission can occur suddenly, often lasting for prolonged periods of time without any discernible reason, which merely adds to the 'mystery' attached to the condition.

Research has not isolated a single common cause. Rather, several issues are known or have been hypothesised, including:

- Metabolic incapacities
- Allergic reaction
- Endocrine disorder
- Toxic elimination
- Central nervous system problems
- Liver impairment
- Gastrointestinal dysfunction
- Autoimmune response
- Heredity

A family history of psoriasis is found in around 30 per cent of cases, a relationship also being drawn between asthmatic forebears and psoriatic offspring, and vice versa. A genetic and therefore hereditary factor adds to the elusiveness of a common 'cure'. In its heritable form, psoriasis can lie 'dormant' until 'appropriate' triggering or provocative factors are introduced. These can range from certain foods to stress and vaccination.

If we accept the heritable factor, psoriasis will only appear in those who are genetically susceptible to it. Indeed, it has been demonstrated that individuals can carry the gene but not have symptomatic expression of it. Studies have identified psoriasis as being latent in individuals with a heritable indisposition.[3]

Psoriatics can be susceptible to arthritis in later years. Between 5 and 10 per cent of us are candidates for psoriatic arthritis, which causes inflammation and stiffness, particularly in the fingers and toes.

Variations of psoriasis

Standard clinical pictures recognise three distinct types of psoriasis according to the size and nature of the individual appearances, namely *guttate*, *nummular* and *pustular*. The commonest form is nummular psoriasis.

GUTTATE PSORIASIS We probably developed this as youngsters. This form occurs mainly in the younger years and often follows a throat infection or some incidence of stress. It is characterised by small scattered spots.

NUMMULAR PSORIASIS This is the commonest and the chronic form, and can develop from guttate psoriasis if it is not properly treated.

FLEXURAL PSORIASIS This is the form which develops under body folds, e.g. in the armpits or the groin. (Also called inverse psoriasis.)

PUSTULAR PSORIASIS (localised and generalised) This sounds pretty horrible and it is, especially in its chronic and inflamed state, where small, sensitive pimple-like eruptions expand, blister and crack with the accompanying dry, scaling and peeling epidermis resembling an eczematous reaction. Small ponds of sterile pus lie beneath the pin-heads. This form afflicts the fingers and palms of the hands and/or the soles of the feet, with or without other types appearing elsewhere on the body.

ERYTHRODERMIC PSORIASIS This red scaly type involves the whole skin and makes fluid and temperature control difficult, which places a considerable strain on the kidneys and heart.

NAIL PITS About one-third of us have nail pits, which is psoriasis under, or of, the nails. Psoriasis on the nails appears as ridging or pitting. Beneath the nails, it causes a yellowing and is clearly noticeable against the normal opaqueness. A severe affliction can cause the nail to distort and crumble, and produce an effect that resembles fungus infection.

Historical research

A skin condition resembling psoriasis is described in ancient medical texts although it is not differentiated from other dermatological conditions. Hippocrates, the Greek physician who lived between 460 and 377 BC, described psoriasis in his notes on diseases, but it was not until the early part of the first century that clinical descriptions were noted in the work of the Roman author, Cornelius Celsus. In *De re medicina*, Celsus described psoriasis as the fourth variant of impetigo (a condition caused by *Staphylococcus pyogenes* and streptococcus infection which manifests in red patches and watery blisters on the skin).

In 1776, Joseph Jacob Plenck (1738–1807) of Vienna wrote of psoriasis in his *Doctrina de morbis*, and described it as being amongst the group of desquamative (scaly or scale-like) diseases, but did not differentiate it further from other dermatological conditions.

Psoriasis was recognised as an independent disease in the work of the

English dermatologist Robert Willan (1757–1812). He categorised the clinical picture of the psoriatic form of skin scaling as *Leprosa graecorum* and the eruptive (exanthematous) form as *Psora leprosa*.

The name 'psoriasis' was first ascribed in 1841 by the Viennese dermatologist Ferdinand Hebra (1816–80), who worked with Willan's notes. He prepared the clinical picture of the disease which is used today. By this time psoriasis was regarded as having a heritable factor.[4]

New developments

The research which has been conducted into psoriasis since the latter part of the twentieth century has produced mostly new and improved ways to describe what was already known, and further elucidated the endocrinal and metabolic factors. Thus the available options for psoriasis treatment have differed little in recent times, whether they be orthodox—variations on gaining symptomatic relief but with possible detrimental effect on the rest of the body, or orthomolecular—an ardent resolve to assist the body heal itself by detoxifying the body and treating a general physiological derangement.

More recently, much excitement has been generated around biotechnology's discoveries with the genome, with several separate and independent announcements of a cure for psoriasis being as little as five years away.

It has been demonstrated how psoriasis could be an autoimmune disease. In this respect, normal immune system response results in abnormal skin cell growth. Under typical conditions an immune response, which is triggered by bacteria, viruses or other factors, calls T cells into action. In some psoriatics who have been studied, T cells which have made their way through the bloodstream to the skin interact with other molecules and cause inflammation.[5] This results in the abnormally rapid rate of skin cell regrowth and the familiar lesions. Biotechnology's strategy for an autoimmune problem such as this is to modify or inhibit the immune system response without causing widespread disruption to cell development.

Elsewhere, antibodies are being developed which could be used to curtail the proliferation of skin cell development and reduce the over-stimulation of capillaries that leads to inflammation.

Meanwhile, perhaps the most significant change is the prevalence of the disease. Our psoriatic numbers must surely be growing in direct relation to our confidence in and persistence with dietary habits which, while commonplace, are nevertheless anti-nutritional and therefore hostile to homeostasis—the body's optimum state of equilibrium or balance. Approximately 250,000 new cases are reported annually in the United States alone.

2 The skin—
an eliminative organ

The skin which envelops your body is actually a body organ. In fact it is an organ ranking with the heart, brain and lungs in its importance to life. While our skins share many characteristics, your skin is unique to you, and mine to me. I wouldn't have it any other way. The skin is:

- A protective organ
- A sense organ
- A regulatory organ
- An absorptive organ
- An eliminating organ

The thickest skin is on the upper back—an average one-eighth of an inch thick—and thinnest on the eyelids—an average one-thirty-second of an inch thick. Your skin is approximately one-sixth of your total weight and contains one-third of all of the blood which is circulating in your body.

The skin comprises two main levels or sections, the epidermis (outer or top layer) and dermis (the layer beneath the epidermis), which is structurally the more complex of the two.

The epidermis, made up of the horny zone (stratum corneum) and the germinative zone, is actually 20 layers of cells (epithelial cells, the layers of skin cells in which there are no blood vessels, and which are also present in the gut wall). The epidermis's deeper layers are bathed in a fluid which is drained away as lymph fluid (see *Figure 1*).

Dead skin cells at the surface of the epidermis disappear daily, through washing and friction. In the lower or Malpighian layer of the epidermis, melanocytes or melanoblasts are busy producing melanin, otherwise this upper level is dormant. Cells in the basal layer of the dermis are constantly renewing and being pushed towards the epidermis in a domino effect, to renew the decaying and shedding cells. The dermis is a hive of chemical activity: sweat and oil glands are hard at work, and the proteins collagen and

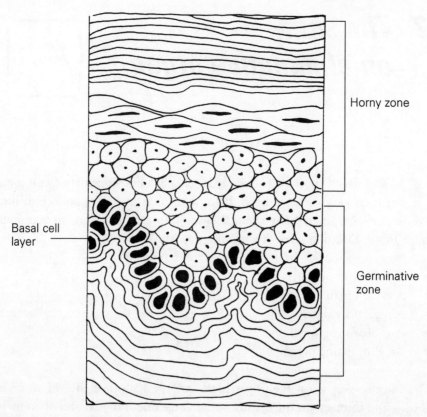

Figure 1: The epidermis

elastin are being manufactured adjacent to hair follicles, nerves and blood vessels. The dermis acts as the chief organ of touch, and secretes sweat and an oily substance (sebum) which prevents too-rapid drying of the epidermis.

Within approximately 0.4 square inch (1 cm²) of skin, we find the following:

- 3 million cells
- 3,000 sensory cells and 200 nerve endings
- 25 pressure touch receptors, 12 sensory receptors for heat and 2 sensory receptors for cold
- 100 sweat glands and 15 sebaceous glands
- 1 yard (1 metre) of blood vessels
- 10 hairs (see *Figure 2*)

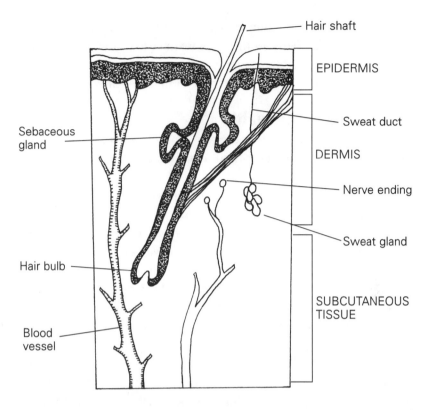

Hair shaft

EPIDERMIS

Sweat duct

DERMIS

Sebaceous gland

Nerve ending

Sweat gland

Hair bulb

SUBCUTANEOUS TISSUE

Blood vessel

Figure 2: The skin

A regulator and filter

The skin is the body's temperature regulator and a storehouse of fats and water, and altogether is composed of many millions of microscopic sensors and glands. It envelops us and acts as the main barrier against harmful organisms and agents (the skin's immune cells, the Langerhans cells, are at the forefront of our body's immune system). It self-manages its blood supply and surface circulation, and regulates our body's interaction with its environment, hence we sweat when the body becomes too hot; gentle greasing by the sebaceous glands is intended to maintain our lustre under drying conditions. Ideal body temperature is maintained at 98.4°F (36°C). The body's temperature might be a little higher in the evening than in the morning.

The skin selectively filters sunlight. It allows some nourishing rays to penetrate, while blocking others to produce pigments, and later provides certain vitamins via the bloodstream to the 'internal body'.

The skin is also a secretionary organ. It relieves overburdened kidneys and lungs of acids and toxins, in the same manner that it will store excess water and salt, or relieve the blood supply and organs of other elements which are likely to become toxic through their overabundance in the system.

Reflection of inner health

The skin can present a true indication of the body's overall condition. As much as one-third of all body impurities are expelled through the skin. It can properly function like this only if it is allowed frequent and regular opportunities to eliminate or release unwanted or excess material through its normal performance. If its eliminatory function is suppressed or disallowed for any reason, an imbalance will occur which invites disease. A diet which contains too much fat, sugar and protein will eventually overwhelm the body's ability to discharge, and ultimately this negative effect will filter through to the skin. Saturated fat and cholesterol will accumulate in the blood vessels and capillaries that service the skin, and deprive it of oxygen and nutrients. A stagnated condition naturally results in restricted elimination.

A diseased skin will not properly function as a forward-line barrier against germs that enter the body; only a healthy skin provides this protection. With diseased skin the entire body's functions are likely to be impaired. This then is further indication that a person with a skin disease deserves careful and thorough internal diagnosis, treatment and constitutional building.

The skin is a vulnerable organ. It can succumb first and proclaim a problem elsewhere in the body system. If the kidneys are damaged, for example, the sweat glands (sebaceous glands) are likely to step in to relieve the body of the waste products that accumulate because of the malfunctioning of the kidneys, or filters. Even under normal conditions the skin acts as an auxiliary excretory organ because the kidneys and skin pores work in harmony with the lungs to remove body wastes.

Pre-programmed for health

Essentially, the skin is programmed for either normal growth or wound healing. Inflamed skin is reddened by increased blood flow to the affected area, which makes the skin feel hot. Swelling results from the body mobilising blood cells that are directed to the area to contain the inflammation and subsequently carry off debris, and the skin feels tender as the result of the irritation of localised nerves caused by the accumulation of fluid and cells. Hives, or urticaria, are an allergic reaction: the histamine released locally into the area causes blood vessels to widen and capillaries to become more permeable, made evident by the characteristic swelling of the skin.

Sebum, sunlight, hormones and hair

Normal healthy skin growth is maintained by sebum, which contains a fatty substance called 7-dehydrocholesterol secreted by the millions of sebaceous glands situated close to hair roots. Sunlight's ultraviolet rays react directly with 7-dehydrocholesterol to produce vitamin D, which is then absorbed into the bloodstream. Through the proper absorption and assimilation of vitamin D into the body system, calcium and phosphorus are utilised and bone tissue is developed and maintained.

Cold conditions congeal sebum and make the skin dry and chapped. Blood flows through the skin more slowly in cold weather than in warm weather, and the reduced nutrient supply results in slower skin growth. Dry skin under temperate conditions arises from an underproduction of sebum. Oily skin results from the overproduction of the lubricant. In adolescence, sex hormones stimulate a rapid increase in sebum production which clogs pores; circulation and excretion are repressed and pimples erupt. The loose wrinkled skin of old age results from de-elasticised skin fibres, caused by decreased sebum production.

Of the two main types of hair, fine hair grows faster than coarse hair. Hair on the scalp is replenished by new growth to the extent of one inch every couple of months. The growth rate of hair on the scalp is not necessarily affected by the presence of psoriasis there. While over 10 per cent of hair is composed of cysteine (a sulphur-rich amino acid), it also contains arsenic, copper, iron, manganese and silica.

Fingernails and toenails

The growth of a 'normal' person's fingernails is approximately two one-hundredths of an inch in one week, which is four times faster than the toenails' growth rate.[1] Blood circulation can influence nail growth (see *Figure 3*).

Life cycle of a skin cell

The skin is constantly shedding old cells, which are replaced with new cells created through cell division. Under normal conditions, the shedding occurs over a period of weeks as the old cells in the epidermis are crowded towards the surface by the creation of new cells below them. This process results from the synchronisation of:

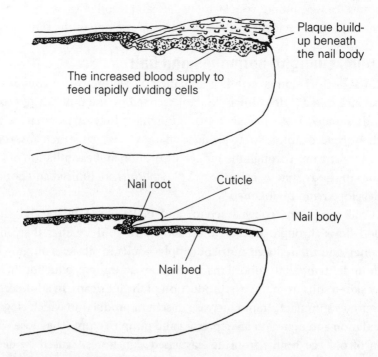

Plaque build-up beneath the nail body

The increased blood supply to feed rapidly dividing cells

Nail root

Cuticle

Nail body

Nail bed

Figure 3: The nail—with and without psoriasis

- Continual cell division in the dermis and the regular supply and maintenance of 'new' cells pushing towards the skin surface;
- Dying-off and shedding of cells (keratinisation); and
- Usually indiscernible de-scaling of the keratinised cells from the surface.

The protoplasm in the cells of the epidermis's horny zone is known as keratin; this zone protects the deeper layer of cells. The keratin cells are constantly cast off by friction, and are replaced by cells from the deeper layers. Normally, keratin cells (keratinocytes) have a 28-day life cycle, which comprises a period of fourteen days when they rise gradually to the surface (epidermis) and a subsequent fourteen-day period when they die and are shed. *In psoriasis, this process takes only two to seven days*. Such a rate of keratinocyte differentiation is too fast to enable the dead keratin cells to be shed in the normal process (which is going on everywhere else on the body where psoriasis is not present) so they accumulate in the form of the familiar plaque (see *Figure 4*).

In this speeded-up activity, the psoriatic condition resembles the way the skin naturally responds to a wound or an infection—the skin cells behave as

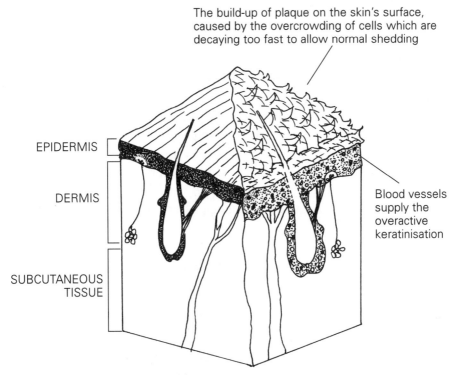

The build-up of plaque on the skin's surface, caused by the overcrowding of cells which are decaying too fast to allow normal shedding

EPIDERMIS

DERMIS

SUBCUTANEOUS TISSUE

Blood vessels supply the overactive keratinisation

Figure 4: Skin / psoriatic skin

if there really is a wound, and switch from their normal growth program to one of vigorous restoration. The rapid cycle results in the build-up of the excess skin cells to form the horny, scaly crust, the white plaque, which covers the psoriatic lesion. The redness revealed when the plaque is peeled away is produced by increased blood supply. Further aggravation or a slight injury to this exposed area can produce a dewy red suppuration.

Pigmentation

In the basal cell layer the melanoblasts contain the pigment melanin. It is melanin, in combination with the nature of the blood supply to the dermis, that gives skin its colour. The amount of melanin present in the basal cell layer varies in races and individuals.

Connective tissue

Under normal conditions, the dermis or 'true skin' is tough, flexible and elastic. It consists largely of collagen (a protein), which is produced when vitamin C converts the amino acid proline into hydroxyproline, and promotes the skin's strength and structure. Collagen makes up 70 per cent of the skin, helps make scar tissue and is damaged by free radicals (see *Chapter 3: Vital Factors in Skin Health*).

External influences

The skin and the central nervous system are intimately interconnected. When drugs are topically introduced (via surface application or injected into the skin) entirely different effects are produced to those which occur when the same drugs are ingested (taken into the bloodstream) or injected under the skin.

The skin is the mirror of the whole body system. Its proper functioning is reliant upon air, light and water to promote circulation, and non-restrictive clothing to promote natural evaporation, respiration and reactions to the environment. Exercise is important for the same reasons, and just as vital as adequate rest. The importance of proper diet is paramount.

Your skin is unique

Because of the skin's relationship with the whole body system—as one of the body's most important eliminating organs—we must regard an ailment of the skin as more than a reaction to internal or external factors. Normal health is impossible unless the skin is healthy. No single organ, or any malfunction or change in a single organ, should be examined without also examining its relationship with the rest of the body. Wholistic medicine takes this a step further, by examining psychological, habitual and personal factors in their relationship to and influence on dis-ease in the individual, recognising that all humans are different and individual in their make-up.

Take care of your skin, the body's largest organ and fourth eliminative organ. It is peculiarly your own and lives and breathes for you alone. In fact, unless it is taken from an identical twin or another part of the same body, transplanted skin will not survive.

3 Vital factors in skin health

There is no one single cause for any degenerative disease, but rather a combination of factors, including the general constitution of the vehicle for disease, the body. The body is programmed to heal itself. We can help it achieve this as willing, active participants in healing. Meanwhile, it is necessary to go back to the basics of how the body works.

The elements of nutrition

A balanced intake of adequate nutrients is essential for everyone, and especially to ensure a strong foundation for gaining control of any disease such as psoriasis. The following nutrients are paramount in the treatment and control of psoriasis and skin disease generally. (The optimum sources for the various nutrients are provided in substantial detail in the tables in Appendix 1.)

VITAMIN A (RETINOL, RETINAL, RETINOIC ACID) Essential for healthy skin, partly because it influences the nutrition of the epithelial cells, and aids against infection by micro-organisms. It is an antioxidant and immune system booster.

VITAMIN B GROUP Each of the B group of vitamins has a symbiotic relationship with a healthy body and skin. The B vitamins listed below have a more direct relationship with psoriasis in particular and healthy skin in general.

VITAMIN B_1 (THIAMINE) An energy producer that also promotes gastrointestinal health.

VITAMIN B_2 (RIBOFLAVIN) Assists in the conversion of fats, sugars and proteins into energy, and the regulation of body acidity; it is essential for repairing and maintaining healthy skin.

VITAMIN B_3 (NIACIN, NICOTINIC ACID, NICOTINAMIDE) Helps balance blood sugar, maintains lower cholesterol levels and promotes digestion.

VITAMIN B_5 (PANTOTHENIC ACID) Maintains a healthy digestive tract and improves the body's resistance to stress.

VITAMIN B_6 (PYRIDOXINE, DECARBOXYLASE) Essential for protein digestion and the utilisation of protein, and helps control allergic responses.

VITAMIN B_{12} Essential for the proper functioning of T cells; it is the only vitamin which contains a mineral element, cobalt.

BIOTIN Helps the body use essential fats and carbohydrates.

BIOFLAVENOIDS Can assist vitamin C with maintaining collagen in healthy condition; this is a comprehensive group which includes antioxidants.

VITAMIN C (ASCORBIC ACID) An important antioxidant and immune system booster which helps turn food into energy.

CALCIUM Activates and regulates digestive enzymes, maintains correct acid-alkaline balance and regulates hormone secretion.

CHOLINE A component of lecithin, choline works in the liver as an aid to breaking down fat, smoothes the movement of fats into cells, and aids the synthesis of cell membranes in the nervous system.

CYSTEINE A sulphur-rich amino acid and an important detoxifier that is essential to the body's proper use of vitamin B_6. Cysteine is effective in addressing imbalances in the metabolising of fats which could otherwise be oxidising and conducive to free radical damage. Over 10 per cent of hair is cysteine.
Note: Diabetics should seek medical advice regarding the use of cysteine.

CYSTINE Similar to cysteine but devoid of antioxidant qualities, this substance is essential to the body's proper use of vitamin B_6.

VITAMIN D (ERGOCALCIFEROL, CHOLECALCIFEROL) Controls calcium and magnesium assimilation, promotes the absorption of calcium from the intestines. (Ergocalciferol is synthetic; cholecalciferol occurs naturally in the body when exposed to sunlight.)

VITAMIN E (D-ALPHA TOCOPHEROL) This is another important antioxidant that helps the body utilise oxygen and improves wound healing.

ESSENTIAL FATTY ACIDS (LINOLEIC ACID, LINOLENIC ACID, ARACHIDONIC ACID) These are polyunsaturated fats that manufacture prostaglandins, the hormone regulators of capillary resistance and blood pressure. They are essential for a healthy immune system as well as healthy skin.

FOLIC ACID (FOLACIN, PTEROLYGLUTAMIC ACID) Essential for utilising protein and facilitates the metabolism of tyrosine and histidine.

GERMANIUM Enriches the body's oxygen supply and activates macrophages (scavenger white blood cells).

INOSITOL (MYOINOSITOL, CYCLOHEXANEHEXOL) Necessary for cell growth; reduces blood cholesterol.

LACTASE This enzyme breaks down the lactose present in cow's milk. If not present in the body lactose intolerance results.

METHIONINE (AMINOMETHYLTHIOBUTYRIC ACID) This precursor to cysteine, cystine and taurine is a free radical forager and therefore useful in detoxification processes. It is essential for promoting the beneficial effects of selenium.

MOLYBDENUM A mineral that plays an important role in helping the body eliminate the waste products (e.g. uric acid, urea and creatinine) which result from protein metabolism. Also an antioxidant.

MUCOPOLYSACCHARIDES These are phytochemicals, long-chain sugars that are constituents of all body tissues and fluids. They are super-powerful antioxidants that bind free radicals on the outside and inside of cells and are effective in tissue regeneration and wound healing. The body's manufacture of these ceases at about age ten.

PHOSPHORUS An essential mineral that helps maintain the body's pH balance, and aids metabolism and energy production.

POTASSIUM Stimulates gut movements to promote proper elimination, maintains fluid balance in the body, promotes the efficient movement of nutrients into cells, and the excretion of waste products from cells.

PROTEOLYTIC ENZYMES These protein-hydrolysing enzymes, which include pepsin and hydrochloric acid, break down food protein into its constituent amino acids.

SELENIUM An essential mineral whose antioxidant properties are useful in protecting against free radicals and in stimulating the immune system; necessary for metabolism; effective with vitamin E in producing antibodies, and can take this vitamin's place in some antioxidant functions such as the protection of cell membranes. Men need more selenium than women; both sexes need its anti-ageing benefits.

ZINC A component of more than 200 enzymes; present in all tissues; aids in coping with stress. It is an important antioxidant and immuno-stimulant.

Metabolism

Metabolism is the complete cycle of changes, both chemical and energy, that takes place in the cells of the body and which is responsible for maintaining growth and repair, and the conversion of complex substances into simpler ones. Disease can be the result of an upset metabolism—the accumulation of waste and toxins in certain cells and tissues in the body can result from faulty metabolism.

Simply put, metabolism is the sum of the way the body deals with nutritive input, the transport of nutrients to aid and regulate cellular activity via respiration and synthesis, and ultimately cell growth and reproduction.

Metabolism occurs simultaneously in two distinct stages: anabolism and katabolism. The former is constructive metabolism, while katabolism is destructive (breaking-down) metabolism. Anabolism uses energy; katabolism usually releases energy. Together these processes produce the glucose which the body requires for energy. The term 'metabolic rate' describes the rate at which metabolic changes occur, measurable by the rate of heat production which ensues from the use of energy which facilitates the chemical changes involved in anabolic and katabolic processes. Nutritional materials (calories) are the source of this energy.

The time of day at which nutrients are taken, the different phases of the metabolic process, and the release of energy which ensues from the breakdown of protein structures, all have a direct relationship with optimum assimilation; thus katabolic nutrients such as protein should be taken between 4 pm and 10 pm. Metabolism is at its slowest between 2 am and 5 am, which coincides with the period when the body temperature is at its lowest; the body is warmest between 2 pm and 5 pm, when metabolism is most active.[1] Enzyme activity reaches maximum capacity when the body is feverish, in symbiosis with the immune functions.[2]

Metabolism also refers to the rate of burning of food substances as fuel in the body, and is measurable by the oxygen that the body consumes in the process. It is influenced by the functioning of the thyroid gland and by diet, particularly in relation to fat and sugar consumption.

One individual's metabolism is not necessarily the same as another's. In addition, different people have different genetically determined requirements for different amounts and types of nutrients. Metabolic typing can be useful in determining individual requirements (see *Part III: Taking Control*).

Psoriasis is associated with at least two problems of metabolism— difficulty in metabolising both the amino acid taurine and the essential vitamin D.

The metabolism of the cells that comprise the skin's inner layer is most active around midnight and slowest twelve hours later, around midday.

The role of enzymes

Absolutely every body function relies upon enzyme action. Enzymes are biological material (chemical compounds, or proteins) produced by living cells that speed up chemical reactions. There are many thousands of enzymes in the human body. They are intrinsic to the essential biological processes that occur in every cell.

Among other things, enzymes prepare the food we eat for absorption into the body, by breaking down large food particles into smaller elements. Specific and well-defined processes, including temperature change, acid-alkali balance, the synergistic presence and/or action of co-enzymes (many related to vitamins, e.g. Q_{10}), inhibitors and other activators are at work in digestion.

Most digestive enzymes control only one reaction, hence the vital importance of proper food combining to promote optimum metabolism and absorption of vital nutrients. Without proper enzyme action our food, no matter how fresh and natural, cannot nourish us. The combination of fats, sugars and proteins in any one meal will also directly influence successful enzyme action.

All enzymes require the presence of moisture; some function in an acid setting, some in neutral conditions, and others in alkaline conditions. They are easily destroyed by, or will not be engaged in the presence of, inappropriate body temperature.

The body relies upon adequate nutrition to enable it to produce sufficient enzymes to properly absorb all food. An enzyme deficiency is a natural flow-on from nutrient deficiency. One such deficiency can result in albinism, caused by the absence of skin pigment.

Any imbalanced condition of the body is further adversely affected by insufficient enzyme activity. The vital factor here is to ensure that enough nutrient-rich food is provided in the diet. Raw food is best, as this not only enables the body to produce more pancreatic enzymes, but is also the source of substantial amounts of other enzymes which aid nutrient absorption. Enzymes in raw foods are activated in the chewing process. Slow, thorough chewing is recommended for maximum results.

Enzymes are secreted by glands; the pancreas is a principal source. Other enzymes are found in saliva from the salivary glands, in gastric juices in the stomach, intestinal juices in the small intestine, and bile in the liver. Enzymes are found only in living things. The enzymes produced for industrial use (for example, in food processing) are derived from animals, plants and micro-organisms. The meat industry is a major provider of these enzymes, from the unused inner organs of slaughtered animals. Rennet, the enzyme vital to the production of cheese, is produced from the stomachs of calves. The purified form of this enzyme is called rennin; children have rennin in their stomachs, whereas adults do not. The benefit of this additional enzyme to the child's metabolism is its ability to curdle milk, which enables the digestion of the protein(s) in milk. Pepsin performs this function in the adult digestive system.

Enzyme production in the body derives from an inherited pattern. Could there be some relationship here between the growing intolerance to 'modern' wheat and the legions of consumers who may be passing on an increased sensitivity?

Enzymes called proteases reduce protein to amino acids. Complex carbohydrates are reduced to simple sugars by amylases (enzymes present in the salivary glands and the pancreas). Fat is turned into fatty acids and glycerol by the digestive juice enzyme lipase.

Cultured and aged foods contain the enzymes protease and amylase. Fermentation has already started the digestive process in such foods—that is, the food is already partially digested and nutrients are more readily available. Aged meats and salamis are such foods. Yoghurt is another.

The enzymes in preserved food (e.g. canned, dried) are largely destroyed by heat and/or preservatives, and thus such foods can be difficult to digest. Many enzymes are susceptible to heating above 118°F (47°C) and cooking destroys them. Conversely, the enzymes in some foods are freed up by cooking—coincidentally, these are good foods for the psoriatic, such as lentils, chick peas and beans.

Acute illness will activate an increase in enzyme levels, providing the body has the necessary resources. However, the reverse is true in chronic conditions, in which enzyme levels drop.

Enzyme deficiency (and/or excess) is implicated in at least 60 diseases. Psoriatics are generally deficient in the enzyme glutathione peroxidase while showing an excess of the enzyme guanyl cyclase. The enzyme lipoxygenase catalyses the formation of inflammatory leukotrienes from the essential fatty acid, arachidonic acid. Garlic and onion and the naturally occurring compound quercetin inhibit the formation of leukotrienes. (The source of any supplemented form of quercetin should be determined, as one version is a by-product of the timber-milling industry and has carcinogenic properties.) While we're on the big words, the enzyme ornithine decarboxylase is also excessively active in the psoriatic. It catalyses the production of polyamines which in turn have a direct relationship with the metabolism of animal protein (see also *Essential Fatty Acids*, page 56, and *Appendix 1*).

Allergies or adverse conditions such as irritable bowel syndrome, the overgrowth of *Candida albicans* and lacto-intolerance can be triggered by digestive enzyme deficiencies. The various enzyme supplements available are discussed in *Part III: Taking Control*.

In body-clock terms, enzymes that break down toxins and ingested drugs are most active around 2 am and at their slowest twelve hours later. It is a fascinating fact that the enzyme charged with the responsibility of breaking down alcohol in the liver has a different timetable in men and women: it is speediest in males at around 8 am, while for females it is doing its hardest work at 3 am.[3]

Protein
Protein is the most plentiful substance in the body after water. All tissues, bones and nerves are comprised mostly of proteins, the major source of

building material. Even scar tissue is formed by a protein, collagen. Protein is active in helping to prevent blood and tissues from becoming either too acid or alkaline, and works with certain minerals to help regulate the body's water balance.

Many psoriatic cases arise from an inborn incapacity to properly metabolise proteins, which allows polyamines (simply, toxins) to accumulate. In some psoriatic cases the amino acid taurine is not properly utilised in the metabolic process.

Protein is required by the body because the life-building amino acids are completely available in complete protein. Amino acids are in fact the chemicals which, when united, form the proteins. The body will synthesise some, but many have to come from food. 'Complete' protein is that which provides at least seventeen of the more than twenty essential amino acids (amino acids are not acids in the popular application). In times of stress or illness, some normally non-essential amino acids (e.g. glutamine) can become 'essential' amino acids. An individual's protein needs are entirely distinctive and are influenced by nutritional condition, body size, age, metabolic type and activity.

Fats and cholesterol

FATS Fats are of three types: triglycerides (found in fats and oils), phospholipids (found in lecithins) and sterols (found in cholesterol, vitamin D and testosterone).

The chemical name for fats is lipids, and they represent the most concentrated form of energy in the diet. Fats have an important role to play in the diet, because when oxidised they provide more than twice the number of calories per gram than carbohydrates or proteins. They assist the absorption of vitamins A, D, E and K, and calcium. The well-known problems with fats arise when there are too many in the diet, or the body is not able to handle their excess because of other attendant malfunctioning. Digestion is prolonged in the presence of fats because they slow down the secretion of hydrochloric acid. No one needs to be told that the prevailing Western diet, with its excess of fast foods, is too high in fats—however, we obviously need to be constantly reminded of it, if the increasing rate of obesity is any indication.

When fats are not completely metabolised they can become toxic in the body. This situation can arise when there is a lack of carbohydrates accompanied by a lack of water in the diet, or there is a kidney malfunction.

Fat in the form of glycogen is stored in the liver and muscles, where it is made available as required through its processing into glucose by enzymes. Fat is also stored under the skin layers and throughout the body, to supplement the liver's reserves.

Fats exhibit different flavours, textures and melting points through the presence of substances called fatty acids. Such differences are obvious in the white fat on a cut of meat and the film that forms on a pot of soup. Body fat is the combination of three fatty acid molecules called triglycerides, attached to a glycerol molecule. How a fat is absorbed in the digestive process is dependent upon its chain length, while the terms 'saturated' and 'unsaturated' reflect the fat's chemical attachments. When certain chemical attachments are missing, such as in most fats derived from plants and fish, the food is described as providing unsaturated fatty acids. The terms 'monounsaturated' and 'polyunsaturated' are applied accordingly to different fatty acids and common characteristics can be identified. Unsaturated (both monounsaturated and polyunsaturated) fats are liquid at room temperature, whereas saturated fatty acids are not—compare vegetable and seed oils with animal fats. Coconut and palm oil, dairy products and eggs also contain saturated fats.

CHOLESTEROL This is a member of the sterol class of fats. There is an ideal cholesterol balance in the body: it is a natural fat-like chemical which is found in many parts of the body and which must be present in a balanced state to promote homeostasis. The brain requires cholesterol, without which it will shrink if it has to deal with chronic alcohol consumption.

Cholesterol is manufactured in the liver, which converts it to bile salts that are essential for digestion and elimination. Cholesterol is required for the manufacture of certain hormones; if there is insufficient cholesterol present in the system the liver will manufacture more. Eighty per cent of the body's cholesterol is produced by the liver and other organs which process carbohydrates, proteins and fats to obtain the compounds essential for cell growth. Cholesterol is a constituent of steroid hormones (the naturally occurring ones), and is converted to vitamin D when the body is exposed to sunlight.

The proper state of digestive bile hinges on the presence of cholesterol, which ensures proper fat metabolism and consequently the adequate absorption of fats and the fat-soluble vitamins (A, D, E and K).

Cholesterol earns its negative reputation partly as a result of being inefficient in its naturally intended role and processes when there is a deficiency of choline, inositol and methionine in the diet. In this state, fat digestion is impaired, other foods are not digested properly, and digestive enzymes have difficulty in reaching food particles through the excess of fat that surrounds them. Animal fats in the diet contribute cholesterol, thereby increasing the total amount in the blood. Problems can arise when cholesterol levels are in excess of basic requirements. As with any fat, cholesterol can be damaged by oxidation and become more difficult to clear from the arteries.

The skin of psoriatics can average 3¼ times the level of cholesterol found in the skin of non-psoriatic persons, a discovery made during research in the United States and published in the November 1950 edition of the *New York Journal of Medicine*.[4] High-cholesterol foods (fatty meats, poultry, liver, brains, shellfish, butter) should be avoided. Lecithin (found in some vegetable oils, nuts, seeds and soybeans) emulsifies cholesterol deposits and also provides choline. Choline is found in egg yolk, along with cholesterol. Eggs are a balanced nutrient source for some metabolic types as they also provide complete protein, iron and minerals. (See *Part III: Taking Control* and *Appendix 1*.)

Carbohydrates

These are energy-providers that require the presence of oxygen to supply the body with calories. Sugar is the most abundant source of carbohydrate. However, sugar is a creature of many faces:

- Monosaccharides: simple sugars such as blood sugar (glucose) and the sugar in fruits (fructose)
- Disaccharides: double sugars such as table sugar (sucrose) and milk sugar (lactose)
- Polysaccharides: complex sugars such as fibre (cellulose) and starches

Of all these, the body can use only glucose to make energy—all other sugars and starches must be converted to glucose by the digestive enzymes. The hormone insulin is critical for the process of metabolising and regulating glucose. Insulin is not needed to convert fructose. This function is completed in the liver for absorption into the blood supply via the intestines.

The body clock

The body has a 24-hour biological clock, known as the circadian biorhythm; each 24-hour phase is a diurnal cycle. This cycle influences how we concentrate and perform basic activities, and regulates many of the body's hormonal activities via the endocrine system, various functions of the sympathetic nervous systems, and our waking and sleeping cycle. The natural rhythms increase prior to dawn, when the appetite is stimulated, heart rate speeds up and blood pressure rises, and hormonal levels increase.[5]

The digestive system

The process of digestion is the sum of the body's systematic physical and chemical actions on food to produce nutrients for itself. It begins with the sense of smell and culminates with the excretion of waste products.

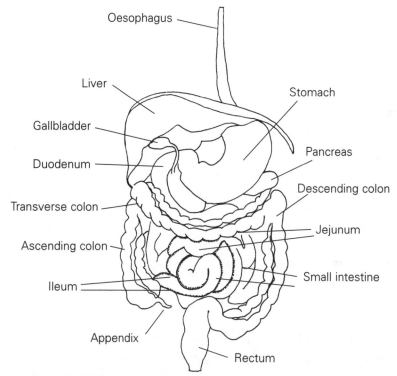

Figure 5: The digestive system

The gastrointestinal tract—the mouth, oesophagus, stomach, small intestine and large intestine (see *Figure 5*)—are all involved in receiving, processing and preparing nutrients which are supplied through a process of absorption from the intestinal tract into the bloodstream. The nature of the prevalent Western diet means that it can take as long as 96 hours for many foods to pass through the digestive tract. A mere four to eight seconds is all it takes for food to reach the stomach after being swallowed.[6] Some foods can remain in the stomach for several hours.

Proteins, fats and carbohydrates require different enzyme actions and stopover times in the stomach. Most enzymes function best in an acid environment, and the digestive juices in general contain the mineral acid hydrochloric acid. Saliva, stomach secretions and intestinal secretions are products of the exocrine glands (as are sweat and tears) which in turn are derivatives of epithelia (surface cells).

Hormones and secretions manufactured in the stomach, duodenum and small intestine act on food to partially digest it, the bacteria in the colon completing the process.

Proteins, fats and carbohydrates are comprised of molecules that are too large for the body to utilise. Of these, protein molecules are the largest and most complex. They must be converted to amino acids, whose molecular structure is sufficiently small to allow their passage into the bloodstream via absorption through the intestinal wall.

The chemical digestion of proteins, carbohydrates and fats follows particular patterns.

Protein (amino acids which are linked in chains)
- Pepsin acts on the food to produce peptones.
- Trypsin and chymotrypsin (juices secreted in the pancreas) act on peptones to produce polypeptides.
- Peptidases (juices secreted in the intestine) act on polypeptides to produce amino acids.

Carbohydrates (starch and sugar)
- Ptyalin (saliva) and amylase (pancreatic juice) work on the polysaccharides (starches) to produce disaccharides (sugars).
- Maltase, lactase and sucrase (intestinal juice) act on disaccharides to produce monosaccharides (glucose).

Fats
- Bile salts (bile) act on fats to produce emulsified fats.
- Lipase (pancreatic and intestinal juice) acts on the emulsified fats to produce fatty acids and glycerol.

The delivery of nutrients into the blood is accomplished via the vascular system (water-soluble nutrients, carbohydrates, lipids and proteins) and the lymphatic system (fat-soluble nutrients in lipids and fat-soluble vitamins). Healthy digestion will provide the body with amino acids, fatty acids, glycerol, monosaccharides, vitamins, minerals and water.

Organs and processes of digestion and absorption

Mouth

- *Dietary fibre* This is the fibre from fruit, vegetables and cereals that remains after the food is digested. Fibre is mixed with saliva to prepare it for swallowing. Within the gastrointestinal tract, the dietary fibre exercises the intestinal walls, with its greatest effect being felt in the colon.
- *Carbohydrates* Salivary amylase begins the digestion of starch to produce polysaccharides and maltose.
- *Fats* Lingual lipase is secreted here, and fats are melted when they reach body temperature.
- *Protein* Chewing prepares the protein food for swallowing.

Stomach

Food is conducted into the stomach by the oesophagus. The gastric juices secreted by glands in the stomach wall to digest the food consist of water, mineral salts, mucus, hydrochloric acid and enzymes.

The digestion of starch begun in the mouth is halted, but the stomach acid partly breaks down maltose and sucrose. The first real step in protein digestion occurs in the stomach, with large proteins being broken down into smaller groups of amino acids.

The release of hydrochloric acid from the stomach wall is dependent upon the presence of zinc, which in turn strengthens the intestinal wall. Both zinc and hydrochloric acid levels diminish with age (a lack of the latter is known to cause allergic reactions, along with the other most common digestive problem in the stomach, a lack of digestive enzymes), hence the body's digestive capabilities diminish with age. Undigested large food molecules, especially the remnants of incompletely processed proteins from a large protein meal, are implicated in indigestion and allergic reactions in the small intestine.

In addition to the production of stomach acid being dependent on the presence of zinc, a lack of zinc diminishes the senses of taste and smell. This can result in a preference for salty and strong-smelling foods, such as cheese and meats, at the expense of fresh vegetables and fruit in the diet.

Acid-forming foods and drinks, and aspirin, irritate the stomach wall, which is experienced as a burning sensation (acid stomach). Aspirin also subverts the metabolism of arachidonic acid.

The stomach is most active between 7 am and 9 am.

- *Dietary fibre* Fibre in the stomach adds bulk to the food.
- *Carbohydrates* Maltose and sucrose are partially broken down by stomach acid.
- *Fats* Acids are mixed with fats and water. Some fat is hydrolysed by the action of gastric lipase, but milk fats are the only fats which are completely digested in the stomach.
- *Protein* Smaller polypeptides result from acid unravelling protein strands. Enzymes are activated.

Small intestine

The small intestine has three parts—the duodenum, jejunum and ileum. The digestion of complex sugars (disaccharides) by alkaline intestinal juices begins in the duodenum. The process of food and beverage digestion introduces approximately 1 gallon (4.5 litres) of water to the body daily. A similar amount of water is added by the small intestine, pancreas and liver. Minerals are absorbed in the small intestine, and calcium is provided along with vitamin D to facilitate the mineral's absorption.

Where non-psoriatic external skin renews itself within three to four weeks, the inner lining of the digestive tract renews itself faster: the stomach cells and mucous membrane of the intestinal tract are replaced every three days.[7]

- *Dietary fibre* Most fibre passes from the small intestine to the large intestine, and beforehand it binds minerals which the body uses to prepare fat for absorption.
- *Carbohydrates* The pancreas releases carbohydrase to break down the polysaccharides to produce maltose.
- *Fats* Fat is emulsified by bile which is supplied by the liver. Monoglycerides, glycerol and fatty acids are prepared for absorption by pancreatic lipase, which breaks down the emulsified fat.
- *Protein* Pancreatic and protease enzymes (supplied by the small intestine) split polypeptides. The peptides are further hydrolysed by enzymes from the intestinal wall's surface which then absorb the amino acids.

Large intestine

The large intestine comprises the colon and rectum (or bowel). In its ascending, transverse and descending formations it is approximately 5 feet

(150 cm) long. Its functions are to reabsorb all possible amounts of water and salt and to store faecal (waste) matter until its expulsion. Here, it is bacteria and not digestive juices which break down the mass.

A diet which is high in fibre, in the presence of a healthy intestinal flora, can speed up the digestive process and prevent the offensive putrefactive odour of faeces.

The rhythmic contraction of the bowel (peristalsis) is reliant upon healthy liver function. If the liver is overloaded, its symbiotic relationship with bowel function will be adversely affected; waste removal will be inefficient and toxins will be absorbed into the blood supply. A strong bowel wall is also essential for clean and strong blood.

The colon is most active between 5 am and 7 am.

- *Dietary fibre* Dietary fibre is relatively undigested by the time it reaches the large intestine where the processing results in glucose ready for absorption. The dietary fibres exercise the intestinal muscles to promote their health and tone. Cholesterol and some minerals are bound with the fibre and duly excreted.
- *Fats* Some fat and cholesterol remain in the faeces.

Liver

The body's most important organ for decontamination, the liver also recycles hormones and is fundamental to the formation of blood. A liver which is disruptive in its functioning might lead to skin disease and can be a cause of psoriasis.

Enzyme production in the liver slows down when the skin temperature falls below 94.2°F (38°C).

Most liver cells have a life span of five months.

Seventy-three per cent of total liver fat is lecithin.

Taurine is used here to convert fat-soluble compounds into water-soluble compounds suitable for excretion.

The liver is most active between 1 am and 3 am.

Pancreas

This is a primary organ of digestion in the breakdown of fats and the release of digestive juices. As a secretory gland it regulates sugar metabolism by releasing insulin into the bloodstream.

The complete process of digestive enzyme production, from the pancreas to their supply to the small intestine, should take approximately 45 minutes.[8]

A diseased pancreas can contribute to skin ailments such as eczema of the anus and urinary tract, as well as fungi in the urinary tract, boils, and abscesses of the sweat glands.

Along with the spleen, the pancreas is most active between 9 am and 11 am.

Spleen
This organ is part of the lymphatic system and is partly formed of lymphatic tissue. It forms antibodies and antitoxins.

Anti-digestion
Sluggish digestion or putrefaction and fermentation in the bowel can cause inflammation leading to degenerative disease.

Fermentation is the opposite of healthy digestion and produces poisons, including acetic acid, carbon dioxide, alcohol, ptomaines and hydrogen sulphide. Bad breath, abdominal gas, foul-smelling stools and abnormal bowel elimination are sure-fire indicators that food is being fermented, not digested. This is an important factor in the incidence of psoriasis and other skin disorders.

Digestion is the process of providing the body with nutrients. The opposite is to create a situation that supports the growth of harmful bacteria. Such an environment can be promoted by incorrect food combining. It can also occur if eating when under stress, angry, anxious, fearful, fatigued, chilled or overheated, feverish, or suffering pain. The level of acidity in the stomach increases when fear releases the hormone adrenalin, while blood flow to the stomach lining is decreased.

Alcohol taken with the meal can also favour the presence of bacterial activity. Over-eating has the effect of expecting the enzyme action to extend beyond its normal capacity. When under stress, the digestive secretions are reduced and blood is shipped off to the muscles. The efficient absorption of nutrients is consequently weakened.

The psoriatic body has several features—it is suffering from a digestive imbalance, probably has a diseased or impaired liver and/or pancreas, and might have an unusually permeable intestine. It is also losing vitamins and minerals through the rapid regeneration of cells and probably suffers from dehydration. The last thing it needs is to exacerbate any problems by missing out on valuable nutrients through faulty digestion. Indeed, the psoriatic would do best to view diet as being paramount in sensible treatment. Anything that reduces or impedes the digestive power and process can be viewed as being antithetic to the body's well-being.

Food combining

One of the culprits leading to an impaired digestive process is injudicious food combining. It is a common error to combine the wrong food types in a meal. Because the individual food types require quite different enzymes and lengths of time for their proper digestion and therefore adequate absorption, it pays to have an understanding of the basic theories and recommended practices of sound food combining.

Starch requires an alkaline medium to be properly broken down and its nutritive qualities maximised via a healthy metabolic process. Protein requires an acid medium. When we eat a carbohydrate, the stomach prepares itself by secreting an appropriate gastric juice. A totally different enzyme is secreted in preparation for the digestion of protein. Even the insertion of a gut probe to measure gut acidity has the effect of changing the ecological acidity.[9]

While the body is intelligent in its response to the need to fine-tune secretions under these circumstances, it is greatly aided by our sensitivity to its basic needs. For example, fruits and proteins, fats and vegetables, are incompatible when combined in the digestive process. Fruits remain in the stomach for only a short time, with most of their digestion taking place in the small intestine. Protein requires a much longer time in the stomach. When protein, carbohydrates and fruits are eaten together, their nutritional value is all but lost; flatulence and the symptoms of digestion warn of possible intestinal dysfunction and disease in the future.

Starch is digested by the salivary secretions, first in the mouth and then in the stomach, where it will remain for a long time if taken under the right conditions or circumstances. If proteins and acids are eaten in combination with the starch, the digestion will be repressed or suspended. The body's digestion of bread, which is a combination of starch and protein, requires two processes. The body will adjust its use of gastric juices, e.g. hydrochloric acid, provided it has a healthy digestive system.

Fruit eaten between meals can lump fructose in with proteins and carbohydrates from a previous meal whilst these are still undergoing their lengthier digestive processes. The rule that accompanies the strictest dissertations on food combining is to eat fruit as a fruit meal. Sugar and protein should not be combined in a meal. Sugars inhibit gastric secretion and the movement of the stomach (gastric motility). Pineapple and papaya contain the protein-digesting enzymes bromelain and papain respectively. Protein combines best with non-starchy vegetables. Beans and peas are a natural combination of starch and protein, and combine with green vegetables.

Fluid taken with the meal will significantly dilute the saliva and weaken the digestive action on starch. It is generally true that drinking water with a meal is not a sound practice, as the enzymes and digestive juices are flushed out of the stomach before they can do their work.

'Leaky gut' syndrome/intestinal permeability

While there are widely variable health pictures associated with psoriasis, the common factors are poor elimination and related intestinal disorders.

The body has four primary routes for eliminating toxins—the skin, lungs, kidneys and colon. We have already noted the skin's role as an eliminative organ. When imbalances in the body reduce the ability of the other organs to do their job properly or there is an overload of toxins in the body system, the body in its continuous need to cleanse will eliminate through the skin.

The wall of the intestine is naturally sieve-like. As a normal process it permits nutrients and other minuscule beneficial compounds to pass through. Blood and lymph circulation carry these to cells throughout the body to do their best. Consider then the role of an intestine that is abnormally 'permeable' (i.e. inefficient because it is irritated or not functioning properly), and which allows the passage into the body system of toxins which otherwise would be adequately dealt with through the normal digestive process. Typical functions would therefore allow blood and lymph circulation to carry these unwanted toxins through the body to do their worst.

The so-called 'leaky gut' syndrome—the condition also called intestinal permeability—arises from irritation or malfunctioning of the mucous membrane of the intestinal wall. The delicate filtering process becomes faulty and permits larger, poisonous particles (read proteins) to escape before they are 'suitably' digested.[10] Excessive amounts of protein can also enter the bloodstream through the assistance of strong alcoholic beverages accompanying a meal.

Intestinal health and permeability can be influenced by many common substances and habits. Aspirin (salicylic acid) irritates the gut wall. For that matter, many of the foods in our diet irritate the very instruments of digestion. Gluten in wheat is such a culprit—but we regard bread as a necessary daily constituent. Gluten is also present in biscuits, cereals, cakes, pasta, noodles and pastries. Baking actually increases gluten's irritating properties. Some treasured fresh foods—fruits and vegetables—also contain salicylates, including tomatoes, a member of the nightshade family, placing them amongst the so-called 'triggers' (see page 71).

The bowel can also develop an uncharacteristic 'leakiness' or excessive permeability. In the instance of an intolerance to cow's milk (lacto-intolerance, i.e. intolerance of milk sugar), the structure of the gut wall is altered by the reaction to the milk and develops a 'leakiness'. The body produces less of the enzyme lactase as we age, which leads to a general propensity for undigested and unabsorbed lactose upsetting our digestive balance. Indeed, the majority of adults are deficient in lactase. Milk also contains at least 20 proteins, amongst them casein and lactalbumin, to which many individuals are intolerant.

Naturally occurring blood cells called eosinophils are implicated in the body's reaction to a protein overload when it is unable to properly deal with the proteins in cow's milk or animal meats. The cells of the stomach and intestinal lining become crowded by eosinophils, with a result similar to intestinal permeability, inasmuch as their presence allows proteins to leak through the bowel wall and into the body system. In this allergic reaction, oedema, especially of the legs, can be a symptomatic result.

A shortage of the essential mineral magnesium can effect histamine release, poisoning from which is evident in symptoms such as skin rashes, headaches and nausea. Intestinal permeability automatically raises susceptibility to histamine poisoning, simply because more can leach through to be taken up in circulation. Histamine is present in foods such as sausages, chocolate and rich cheeses.

Antibiotics, including tetracycline which is often prescribed to treat acne by inhibiting bacterial growth, also kill friendly intestinal bacteria and lay open the way for leaky gut and candida.

Intestinal permeability is linked to various health problems, including reactive arthritis, allergies and autoimmune joint diseases.

Should you find that you possess this leaky gut syndrome, its treatment is quite straightforward. The application of suggestions contained in *Part III: Taking Control*, principally those referring to dietary and herbal treatments, have been effective in correcting such disturbances. Obtain the assistance and advice of a practitioner who is qualified and able to identify and confirm the presence of the intestinal weakness so described. It is also important to consider the likely role of your gut's dislike for cow's milk.

Intestinal permeability as a principal factor in psoriasis was described 70 years ago by Edgar Cayce (1877–1945), the seer better known for his 'readings' provided via a hypnotic sleep state. At an early age, Cayce mastered his school lessons by sleeping on his textbooks. At age 21, a throat paralysis threatened the loss of his voice. By entering the sleep state, he was able to recommend a cure which repaired his throat muscles and restored his voice.

On numerous occasions thereafter, he recommended treatments and cures for many conditions. For most of his life, Edgar Cayce provided intuitive insights into a very broad range of questions about medical problems. His psychic readings also concerned business planning, meditation, dreams and prophecy, with the body of his work comprising over 14,000 readings on more than 10,000 different topics.

Importantly for us, Cayce offered invaluable insight into the incidence and treatment of psoriasis. He was quite explicit about the role of the lymphatic system and the area of the upper small intestine between the duodenum and the jejunum (see *Figure 6*), and recommended the abolition of red meat, fried foods, alcohol and carbonated beverages from the diet.

Cayce was also able to prescribe treatments to achieve remission in cases of psoriasis, which were characteristically simple and straightforward, namely:

- Internal cleansing (detoxification)
- Healing of the intestines
- Diet and nutrition

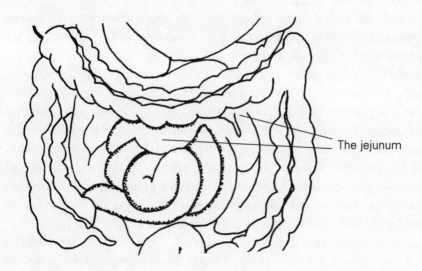

The jejunum

Figure 6: The jejunum

- Spinal adjustment
- Attitudes and emotions

Note, however, that Cayce's readings were given for individuals; he did not attribute all cases of psoriasis to intestinal problems.[11]

Dr John O. A. Pagano, a chiropractor, has written at length on his work with psoriatics using the Cayce treatment methodology with much success. Dr Pagano also found that certain plants of the nightshade family were amongst the triggers for psoriasis.[12]

The application of osteopathy or chiropractic to achieve spinal adjustment is interesting. Cayce identified problems with the vertebrae as one of the primary causes of the permeable intestinal wall. Pressures on spinal nerves, particularly in the mid-dorsal area, can adversely affect the transmission of nerve energy to the intestines. Adjustments to correct this misalignment can improve nerve system function.[13] Two studies by the Meridian Institute testing Cayce's treatment recommendations confirmed the evidence in his readings and in Dr Pagano's clinical work, although a few participants in the studies experienced little improvement in their psoriasis.[14]

Intestinal yeast and bacteria

Gut yeast has been found to have a role in psoriasis. *Candida albicans* is one such yeast. If it is present in overload quantities, the psoriatic's body has a multiplicity of factors to deal with, including a damaged bowel wall. If yeast infection is overwhelming, the body will become toxic. *Candida albicans* is a yeast-like fungus which occurs most commonly in the digestive tract and vagina, and which can harbour over 70 different toxic products. Thrush and yeast infections are its symptoms.

The 'friendly' intestinal bacteria, *Bifidobacteria* and *Lactobacillus acidophilus*, are foremost in the detoxification process. They not only help to digest food, but also stimulate normal peristaltic action (the rhythmic contracting and relaxing which moves the contents along the intestine). Adversely affected by antibiotics, these bacteria are necessary for controlling undesirable bowel residents such as candida. They are also adversely affected by diets that are too high in fat, red meat and sugar.

Food intolerance could result from these beneficial bacteria becoming disturbed and less abundant, which invites infestation by harmful bacteria. The harmful bacteria feed on the chemicals produced by some foods and thereby provoke the 'symptoms'.

In the presence of enzyme defects and/or a lack of certain detoxifying enzymes, an already disturbed gut flora can be worsened and create symptoms of food intolerance. The environment can also be made more susceptible to damaging bacteria such as candida.

Essential fatty acids

The three classifications of fat—saturated, unsaturated and poly-unsaturated—describe the stability of their chemical bonds. All fats and oils are made up of fatty acids—building blocks in a balanced body system. They provide more than energy.

The body requires certain types of fat in order to be healthy. They are essential to the efficient breakdown and transport of cholesterol, and in general terms are necessary for normal growth and the health of nerves, arteries and blood. Polyunsaturated fatty acids can all be synthesised from a diet of protein, carbohydrates and fats, with the exception of the essential fatty acids, which cannot be made by the body. It is therefore reliant upon their provision in the diet. The essential fatty acids are linoleic acid (omega-6), alpha-linolenic acid (omega-3) and arachidonic acid.[15]

The body produces important derivatives from these—GLA, DGLA, AA, EPA and DHA—and prostaglandins, which are hormone-like substances found in seminal fluid and to a lesser extent in the kidneys, lungs, brain and other tissues. Essentially, GLA et al play an important role in the body's circulatory system, and in haemoglobin production, immunity, brain function, and cell division and respiration. They are carriers of vitamins A, D, E and K, are closely linked to the health of skin, nails and hair, and help break up cholesterol in the bloodstream.

Sufficient levels of omega-6 can reduce cravings for fatty foods in general. Omega-3 can be destroyed by cooking and other food processing methods. When unstable fatty acids are damaged in these ways, they can bond with oxygen atoms and become free radicals, which damage cells in the absence of sufficient antioxidants in our body system and diet. Vitamins C and E are antioxidants that our body system requires to deal with these free radicals. All living cells contain antioxidants, and they are provided to some degree in all foods.

Amino acids

Protein is made from amino acids through their joining together into chains. Children have a slightly different need of amino acids to adults, and every individual has a different optimum requirement for amino acids (as with all other nutrients, for that matter). There are more than 20 essential amino acids—essential because they are required for the development of other amino acids and the proteins required by the body. If one essential amino acid is not present, or is present in too low an amount, protein synthesis will fall to a very low level or cease altogether. Amino acids are composed of a combination of carbon, hydrogen, oxygen, nitrogen and sometimes sulphur. Foods such as meats, fish, poultry and dairy are high in protein and provide a good proportion of amino acids. Spirulina is a fine natural source.

The eight essential amino acids are isoleucine, leucine, lysine, methionine, phenylalanine, threonine, tryptophan and valine.

An adequate intake of essential and non-essential amino acids is also important to ensure synthesis of certain metabolic products, including taurine (synthesised from cysteine) and melanin (the skin and hair pigment). Melanin is synthesised from tyrosine and is produced by pigment cells. Hormonal and neural factors influence melanin synthesis.

Taurine, a neurotransmitter, is of significance amongst the (non-essential) amino acids through its direct relationship with psoriasis. Research by nutritional scientist and dermatologist of Cornell University, USA, Dr D. Roe, highlighted psoriatics' incapacity to properly metabolise taurine (and the losses of nutrients in psoriatics, even those with adequate dietary intake).[16]

Taurine (with aspartic and methionine) is a katabolic amino acid and is needed for the correct composition of bile. It is present in large amounts in all types of protein, and is an additive in infant formulas. As a component of specific bile acids, taurine aids the digestion and absorption of lipids such as cholesterol in the gastrointestinal tract. The liver uses taurine to convert fat-soluble compounds (e.g. lipids) into water-soluble complexes that the body ultimately excretes. The formation of taurine in the liver is repressed by estradiol, the female hormone.[17]

Proper balancing of the mineral salts sodium and potassium is assisted by the presence of taurine. It smoothes the progress of calcium, magnesium, sodium and potassium ions in and out of cells.

As a katabolic amino acid, taurine is active at different phases in the metabolic process. It is important to understand how these processes are active at certain times of the day. (See also *Table 3* in *Appendix 1*.)

Acidity (of the blood)

This term actually refers to a condition of reduced blood alkalinity. In fact life would be impossible if the blood reached an actual acidity. Its use here refers to a condition of imperfect elimination and a diet imbalanced in favour of acid-forming foods.

During normal metabolism, acids are continually being formed, decomposed and eliminated through the kidneys, skin, lungs and bowels. Other acids (such as uric, oxalic and oxybutric acids, and acetones) are often introduced with foods. When they are not eliminated or are taken in excessive amounts, their accumulation results in acidity of the blood or toxaemia.

Alkalinising or neutralising foods should be substituted for acid-forming foods. Fats, proteins and all rich foods should be omitted from, or at the very least reduced in, the diet. Thorough bowel elimination and exercise to stimulate the circulation are essential to achieve a reversal of the acidic blood state. (See also *Acid-forming and alkaline-forming foods* in *Part III: Taking Control, pages 162–163*.)

Toxaemia

This term refers to toxins in the blood, which if unchecked can result in disorders affecting the skin and mucous membranes, digestive diseases, bronchitis and catarrh. For example, an accumulation of uric acid can lead to inflammatory conditions such as gout. Alcohol, caffeine and chocolate stimulate the production of uric acid. Purines also stimulate the production of uric acid. These substances are found in shellfish, anchovies, sardines, mussels, herrings, mushrooms, meat gravies and stocks, as well as yeast products, oatmeal and baked goods.

All vital organs work hard in the ongoing detoxification process to eliminate harmful substances. Poor elimination and sluggish bowel conditions—leading to intestinal toxaemia or leaky gut—can be caused or exacerbated by a lack of beneficial bacteria in the gut. Chlorinated water, chemical pollution and antibiotics all are detrimental to these bacteria.

Effective elimination and building-up of the constitution are the obvious courses for treatment, together with specialised attention to the whole body system.

Toxification

Psoriasis will not respond positively to nutritional intervention alone, unlike eczema and dermatitis which should respond to diet, given the appropriate direction and a firm commitment. Nevertheless, considering the very real likelihood of toxification of the body, the indisposition of the liver in the detoxification process and therefore digestive imbalances, there is genuine cause to address the diet in cases of psoriasis. Especially necessary is to avoid, or significantly reduce, dairy products and meat, and to increase the intake of essential oils from natural sources.

Blood health

A healthy blood supply's relationship with the immune system is critical. The white blood cells are the 'cleaners' and therefore the mainstays in immune system response and day-to-day body maintenance. They are comprised of granulocytes, the most common of which are the neutrophils, and non-granulated cells (monocytes and lymphocytes). Neutrophils do not need an immune system 'invitation' from damaged tissues, but instead migrate of their own volition. They can be witnessed in their 'cleaning' up of plasma in the blood of a person whose immune system is strong, and whose blood supply is consequently also healthy and strong.

In the naturally occurring immune process called phagocytosis, the neutrophil draws the offending bacterium into itself and systematically breaks it down until it is finally destroyed. Monocytes follow on from neutrophils, and on entering the tissue swell to many times their original size, when they become macrophages.

Secondary to the neutrophils are the lymphocytes (thought to derive from bone marrow, lymph tissue and the spleen) and, in lesser numbers still, the eosinophils. Lymphocytes produce antibodies in their function as a major player in cellular immunity. Eosinophils' numbers are generally low in normal loose connective tissue, but they figure enormously in response to inflammatory and allergenic reactions (the state known as eosinophilia).

Blood purity is directly related to bowel condition. If the bowel is in poor health, the blood will be sticky and dirty, and the neutrophils will be sluggish in their work.

Free radicals

Actually 'free oxidising radicals', to give them their full title, these foraging cell-damaging entities and the precursors of disease are toxic substances that are created through the oxidising of molecules by unstable oxygen, and which are present in the bloodstream or tissues. Free radicals in the form of waste products that result from normal metabolism or stress are particularly relevant to psoriasis. However, everyone is susceptible to damage from free radicals that are not dealt with by adequate antioxidant action. Free radicals are actually endeavouring to achieve stability, and in this process latch onto and tear into neighbouring stable molecules. This can set off a chain reaction, with cumulative molecular and structural damage.

There are two main types of free radicals (hydroxyl and superoxide). They arise from all forms of combustion and are present in sources as diverse as fried and burnt foods, pollution, fuel combustion and normal body functions. Our modern world also provides free radicals in toxic industrial chemicals, ionising radiation, pesticides, food additives, cigarette smoke and drugs. They can also originate in artificial and natural ultraviolet light, and be produced by high-intensity exercise and stress. The body also produces free radicals as a part of normal metabolic processes. For example, the liver uses free radicals which it produces to break down toxins; phagocytes (cells which gobble up other cells and micro-organisms as a part of the naturally occurring immune process) use free radicals. Phagocytes carry a large amount of taurine, which is present in its antioxidant state, to protect themselves from cytotoxic substances. Cumulative problems can result if an imbalance favours the free radicals, or when the body does not possess sufficient antioxidants (free radical destroyers) to deal with the harmful scavengers. Thus a consistent fresh supply of antioxidants is essential to health.

Leaky gut syndrome presents an environment encouraging free-radical damage, because of the seepage of toxins through the intestinal wall into the body system. While this is a natural occurrence to a degree under normal body conditions, the psoriatic's general indisposition invites greater susceptibility, with or without the abnormally permeable intestinal wall that characterises leaky gut syndrome.

Melatonin, which is produced in the pineal gland, destroys free radicals with great efficiency. Its secretion peaks in childhood and lessens as we get older. Reduced melatonin levels are implicated in degenerative diseases.

Overall, free radicals' natural balancing factor is the antioxidants, chief amongst which are the body's enzymes, superoxide dismutase and glutathione peroxidase. Vitamins A, C and E, and beta-carotene, the precursor to vitamin A, are essential antioxidants, as is selenium, on whose presence glutathione peroxidase depends. There are also hundreds of other non-essential nutrients which provide antioxidants, in the form of bioflavenoids, for example. (See *Chapter 7: Internally—Nutrition for Skin Health* and *Appendix 1*.)

The endocrine system

The ductless endocrine system (see *Figure 7*) is the chemical control centre of the body. It is composed of eight glands:

- Pineal
- Pituitary
- Parathyroids

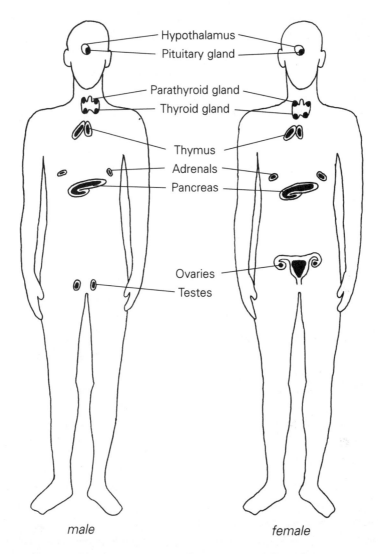

male *female*

Figure 7: The endocrine system in the male and female

- Thyroid
- Thymus (which controls the immune system)
- Adrenals
- Pancreas
- The reproductive glands (female ovaries and male testes).

The adrenals, pineal and thyroid are elaborated on below.

The endocrine system's chemicals are the hormones, which are secreted directly into the bloodstream. Their proper balance is essential for life; they have a fundamental role to play in metabolism, control bodily, intellectual and emotional growth, and influence sexual development and function. The thyroid hormone and insulin (from the pancreas) are proteins.

The adrenals produce more than 40 hormones, the most significant of which are members of the cortisone family. Steroid drugs are their synthetic analogues.

Amongst the hormones are the neurotransmitters serotonin, dopamine, adrenalin and acetylcholine, all biochemical messengers in the nervous system. They differ from the non-neurotransmitter hormones in that they carry nerve impulses from the brain, using cell membranes throughout the body. The immune system sends its messages via the neurotransmitters called cytokines.

A low serotonin level is implicated in violent behaviour. Serotonin is widely distributed in body tissue, in the gastrointestinal lining (where it stimulates involuntary muscle in the intestinal wall), in blood platelets and in the brain. Alcohol, stress, low levels of melatonin and artificial electromagnetic fields are known to suppress serotonin, which is widely used in the treatment of depression. The amino acid tryptophan is converted in the body into serotonin.

Hormone activity is at its peak between 7 am and 9 am.

Adrenal glands

The adrenal gland has two parts—the adrenal and supradrenal, also known as the cortex and medulla. They secrete the hormones adrenalin and noradrenalin. Adrenalin, secreted by the medulla, is necessary for overcoming sudden stressful conditions. It prepares the body for emergency response by speeding up the pulse and diverting blood to the muscles from the intestines and the skin. An immediate supply of energy results from the conversion of glycogen in the liver into glucose.

Pantothenic acid is necessary for the synthesis of adrenalin (as are cholesterol and fats), and in symbiotic relationship with the adrenal cortex produces cortisone and other adrenal hormones which are important for healthy skin and nerves. Undealt-with stress will deplete the body's levels of pantothenic acid and other B vitamins. (See also *Table 6* in *Appendix 1*.)

Black coffee poured into an empty stomach will vigorously activate the production of adrenalin, giving somewhat more than the familiar 'rush'. The 'common office environment', characterised by competition for promotion and 'proactively' achieving 'targets' on behalf of 'stakeholders' as a member of a 'team', the stress these experiences engender, and the ubiquitous coffee machine and proliferation of high-caffeine 'energy' drinks, do not augur well for optimum adrenal synthesis.

Thyroid gland

This gland regulates bodily growth and activity through the secretion of hormones.

Metabolism is controlled by the thyroid hormones as is the level of calcium in the blood which is essential to the proper development of bones. Calcitriol, which is produced by the kidneys from vitamin D, is an essential part of this process.

A body's inability to deal with animal protein is exacerbated in cases of hypothyroidism (i.e. underactive thyroid hormone secretion).

Pineal gland

This gland, located deep within the brain's centre, produces melatonin. The synthesis of this hormone, which is critical to numerous body systems and functions, not the least of which is the production of the neurotransmitter serotonin, is prominent at night. Melatonin's secretion decreases with age, and is present in lesser levels in people over the age of 60 years. It has been used to enhance moods, and induces a feeling of well-being and comfort. Melatonin production can be adversely effected by electromagnetic frequencies which are not much greater than the earth's natural magnetic background (such as those which emanate from normal ambient household appliances, electric blankets and waterbeds.)

The lymphatic system

The lymphatic system of vessels and glands stems from the circulatory (blood) system and eventually passes back into it (see *Figure 8*). Unlike the bloodstream, which is pumped through the body by the heart, the lymph system relies on exercise as the driving force for stimulation and circulation. Deep breathing, massage and non-stressful physical exercise are very beneficial to lymphatic circulation.

The lymphatic system is another important filtering system. It permeates the skin and the tissues over the entire body, with lymph nodes to trap and filter harmful organisms, cell debris and foreign matter. It is these nodes which become inflamed, such as those in the neck which swell with a throat infection or cold. However, the familiar soreness or sensitivity to touch is not caused by the nodes becoming clogged with harmful bacteria. The swelling

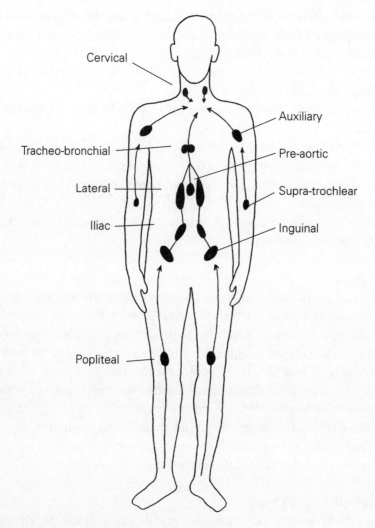

Figure 8: The principal lymphatic glands

results from the marshalling of blood cells to deal with invasive infection, thus we are afforded a clear warning that the body is harbouring unwanted bacteria and that it is time to take preventative measures. The nodes also manufacture and store the immune function agents, the lymphocytes and macrophages, which protect against toxicity, infection and cancer.

Lymph is the medium by which oxygen and nutrient substances (vital proteins) in the bloodstream are delivered to the tissues, and which removes waste products from the blood supply. The epidermis's deeper layers are well serviced by a fluid which is drained away as lymph.

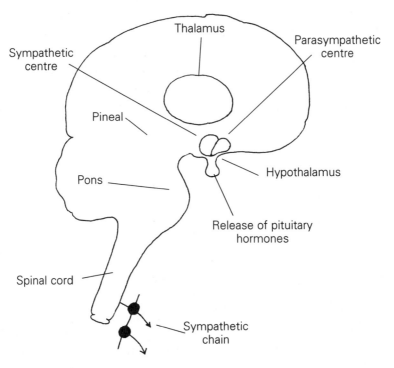

Figure 9: The brain

A diet which is overloaded with toxins will tax the lymphatic system and invite blockages. Conversely, good nutrition will enhance lymphatic action and drainage, and promote optimum metabolism.

The autonomic nervous system

The autonomic nervous system controls the body's internal functions. It is comprised of the sympathetic nervous system and the parasympathetic nervous system (see *Figure 9*). They are stimulated by multiple brain centres that are located in the hypothalamus and the brain stem.

The hypothalamus is of immense importance, as it has direct influence on physical and emotional states. It is the control centre for the regulation of the immune system, the cycles of sleeping and waking, emotion, neuro-endocrine functions, and calorie intake. Amongst the neurotransmitters at work here is glutamate.

The significance to the psoriatic of the sympathetic and parasympathetic nervous systems is their influential relationship with gastrointestinal movement and health. For example, parasympathetic stimulation increases peristalsis and plays a key role in the exocrine system's control of the secretion of digestive juices via some of the glands in the gastrointestinal tract, the salivary glands and the gastric glands. Food can pass from the mouth to the anus within approximately 30 minutes under extreme parasympathetic stimulation, whereas the normal transmission time is about 24 hours. However, sympathetic stimulation has the reverse effect of inhibiting peristalsis, thereby slowing the movement of food through the gastro-intestinal tract.

The metabolism of all of the cells of the body is increased under generalised sympathetic nervous system stimulation.

The central nervous system

The central nervous system (CNS) is the body's electrical system—it functions through minute impulses of electrical energy. Cell division is an electrical process, enzymes are chemical messengers which enlighten the body organism. Without the CNS and its chain of neurones the body would not know what to do. It regulates directly in accordance with the body's needs.

The CNS (brain, spinal cord and peripheral nerves) is composed of the peripheral and autonomic nervous systems. The brain is at the pinnacle of the nervous system. Its chemical messengers, together called neuropeptides and peptides, are the myriad complex chemical substances which it secretes—hormones, neurotransmitters and the opiate-like endorphins. These messengers have free passage throughout the body, and as emissaries of the brain, carry very definite signals that are capable of instructing, activating, and regulating our immune system.

The amino acid taurine is present in the central nervous system.

Phosphatidyl choline, a phospholipid, is fundamental to healthy nerve system function, the control of sensory input signals and muscular control. A deficiency of choline can be apparent in poor memory, lethargy and a decrease in dreaming, and result in fatty deposits in the liver.

The limbic system

While the entire nervous system affects one's behaviour, it is the limbic system which controls involuntary aspects of behaviour, and is central to the excitation of pain and pleasure, anger and fear. It is centred on the limbic cortex, a specific ring of the brain's cerebral cortex known to be amongst the earliest parts to have evolved in primitive animals.

The hypothalamus is central to the limbic system's influence on behaviour, its input deriving from the thalamus, hippocampus and amygdala. The limbic system thus works through the autonomic nervous system. It also works through the endocrine system, via the appropriation of pituitary hormones, to exercise significant influence on day-to-day cellular metabolic functions.

Because of its inherent role in behaviour, the limbic system has an influence on one's inner being, and a direct relationship with the development and recognition of thought. The limbic system employs information 'remembered' from past experiences, which it uses to initiate behavioural responses, including emotions.

The blood–brain barrier

This is a cellular wall comprised of capillaries whose primary purpose is to prevent toxic substances from entering the brain. However, not all toxic substances are prevented from entry, as has been discovered in research into excitotoxins cited by Russell L. Blaylock, MD, in *Medical Sentinel* (see Excitotoxins, pages 76–77). Free radicals are also capable of penetrating the blood–brain barrier.

Within the brain, the hypothalamus and pineal gland in the circumventricular organs are not protected by the barrier system. This lays them open and susceptible to neurotoxins, amongst the worst of which are manufactured glutamates and aspartates. The barrier is eroded by chemotherapy and some drugs, and the natural process of ageing also reduces the barrier's effectiveness. Certain diseases also dispose sufferers to a permeable blood–brain barrier. These include diabetes, multiple sclerosis and hypertension.

The immune system

Our immune system is a brilliant mechanism. Essentially it is working well when it is allowed to maintain balance. Cooperation amongst diverse brain and body mechanisms and cells is intrinsic to healthy immune system function; therefore an alert and successful immune system is aided by and dependent upon properly functioning blood circulation, a healthy CNS, hormonal balances, a strong digestive system, and an alert and positive mental attitude. By proxy all of these are part of the immune system.

The healthy immune system activates the production of antibodies that are specific to antigens which threaten imbalance. Protein molecules from animals are amongst such antigens (which also include polysaccharides) and pollen from plants and flowers. Simple allergies to pollen, dust, moulds and foods will trigger a familiar immune system reaction.[18] Having once overcome an intruder which threatens imbalance, the immune system remembers the 'key', so that the body will quickly recognise and pre-empt a problem before it arises next time. When the body is sick, extra white blood cells are released from the thymus, spleen, tonsils, appendix and lymph glands to boost the working of the immune system.

Gut microbes are kept where they belong—in the gut—by a healthy immune system. In coeliac disease (a disease of the small intestine characterised by gluten intolerance), a broad theoretical explanation has the antibodies created by the immune system causing damage to the gut wall in its response to perceived unwanted substances.[19]

In its healthy state of preparedness, our immune system allows fully digested food to pass through the gut wall into the body, to do its nourishing best (provided the food we eat is truly nourishing). The immune system regards amino acids, fatty acids and some sugars as partners in this process.

High levels of endorphins have an inextricable relationship with a healthy immune system. These are the anti-stress hormones which also figure in natural pain relief. They are boosted by positive emotion and enjoyable experience—laughing out loud, making love, stress-free exercise—by antioxidants, and fresh fruit and vegetables. They are worn away by undealt-with stress, negative emotions and thoughts, and extreme fatigue, chronic pain and illness.

Significantly, too, the immune system is itself capable of producing peptides, which are transmitted back to the CNS.

Immune cells

There are three types of immune cells, all of which originate in bone marrow stem cell—the T cells, B cells, and granulocytes and monocytes.

T cells or T lymphocytes mature in the thymus gland, and are comprised of T helpers, T suppressors, and NK (natural killers). B cells mature from the spleen and other organs and produce plasma cells. The white blood cells—granulocytes (which mature as basophils, mast cells and neutrophils) and monocytes (which develop into macrophages)—patrol the body as primary agents in the immune system's protective role. They destroy and eliminate dead red blood cells and are capable of attacking bacteria, including those which the body does not possess antibodies against.

There is some conjecture as to the number of T cells that are produced, due to the lifetime of the thymus gland. It has been held for some time that they are produced only in the first few years of life, after which the thymus gland shrinks and shuts down, presumably having provided the body with a lifetime's supply of T cells. They diminish in number with age, and consequently the body's ability to fight bacteria and viruses also slows down.

Others, notably professor of genetics David Suzuki, suggest that a certain level of production of T cells might continue in the lymph glands.[20] The thymus gland's production of T cells is stimulated by peptides emanating from the hypothalamus and pituitary gland.

According to some researchers, psoriasis is a T cell-initiated disease. Activated T cells were discovered to be present in psoriasis lesions, and furthermore they were releasing inflammatory proteins,[21] which were found to be the cause of the overgrowth of the skin cells in the psoriasis lesions. Overgrowth equals the death of skin cells and this, together with the inflammation, was correlated with the presence of T cells. This research figured in an overall program that centred on treatment of disease by manipulating the immune system.[22]

Melatonin has been found to enhance T cells. T cell counts can be increased and the T helper:suppressor ratio improved by gentle exercise and activity such as meditation and tai chi, whereas vigorous exercise can actually suppress the immune system.[23]

Genes and heredity

Presumably anyone can develop psoriasis. The assumption that psoriasis is hereditary arises from the first-family association in one out of every three cases recorded, although so far there is no one defined pattern of inheritance from one to subsequent generations.[24] Under this theory, one gene modified by others in combination with environmental factors produces the disease. In other words, the gene can lie dormant until a triggering agent sets off the chain reaction which results in psoriasis plaques on the skin surface.

Genes control heredity from parents to children. A gene is a hereditary 'word', if you like—a complete set of genes is the genome, or 'dictionary'. All organisms contain cells which contain complete sets of genes, and therefore genomes.

Many genes can be constructed with 100 to 1,000 'letters', but rather than these hereditary words having a single meaning, they can contain virtual chapters of information. A human being's genetic code may carry a million of these 'words'. A human cell's genome contains 23 chromosomes. Each of these is comprised of two DNA molecules bound together in the famous double helix. Each of these molecules represents our one million genes, which in turn are comprised of 'base pairs'. It is through configurations of base pairs that the 'message of heredity' is conveyed, or an alphabet of heredity constructed, by which it is possible to translate the meaning of the gene.

Homo sapiens and the higher plants and animals each have 46 chromosomes (as 23 pairs). These chromosomes, and the information they contain which dictate an individual's existence, are present at conception. The measured effects of radiation poisoning and some diseases establish that chromosomes are susceptible to damage. It will be postulated elsewhere in this book that genetic alphabets—or hereditary factors—may be self-altered.

Genes not only control heredity from parents to children, they also control the day-to-day function of all cells. Genes determine the enzymes and chemicals that will be synthesised within the cell, and the cell's structure. Each gene is a nucleic acid (deoxyribonucleic acid, or DNA), which controls the formation of another acid (ribonucleic acid, or RNA). The formation of a specific protein is controlled by the RNA spreading throughout the cell.

A normal human body contains cells that are growing and reproducing all the time, controlled by the genetic mechanism. Replication of the DNA is the first stage in cell reproduction—the formation of a duplicate set of cells. This leads to the replication of all the chromosomes in the cell. Once a complete new set of chromosomes has been formed, cell mitosis produces two new offspring cells. Some cells are growing and reproducing constantly, notably the germinal layers of the skin and the epithelium of the gut, together with the blood-forming cells of bone marrow, whereas the neurons and striated muscle cells do not reproduce at all. The body modifies cell reproduction to cope with cell insufficiencies. For example, cells of the subcutaneous tissue and the epithelium of the intestines grow and reproduce rapidly until the appropriate numbers are available. This process is supported by control substances called chalones, which are secreted in the different cells and monitor and effect responses to slow or stop cell growth and reproduction.

Psychosomatic factors

When one is told that psoriasis is a psychosomatic disease, the suggestion is being made that the bodily (somatic) effect is produced by psychological stimulation. Not so long ago several common diseases were regarded as having purely psychological origins. They included neurodermatitis, high blood pressure, hyperthyroidism, rheumatoid arthritis and ulcerative colitis.

It is erroneous to infer that a psychosomatic disease is in some way a hypochondriacal invention. Because of the physiological functions of the brain in partnership with the autonomic nervous system, our thoughts, memories and emotions can trigger disease. A typical physiological response to a psychosomatic inducement brings into play the autonomic nervous system, and the stimulation of thalamus or hypothalamus. Psychosomatic effects can cause individual organs to function abnormally. Gastrointestinal activity can be so decreased by the activity of the sympathetic nervous system that constipation results; an overly active parasympathetic nervous system can cause diarrhoea. Emotional conditions can give rise to peptic ulcer (another of the diseases formerly held to be of purely psychological origin). This arises through the stimulation of the parasympathetics that control gastric juice secretion in the stomach. These can become so over-stimulated, and the juice secretion so extreme, as to cause a hole to be eaten away in the gut wall or upper intestine.

Sympathetic activity caused by fear, anxiety or fury will course throughout the body and stimulate organs. Parasympathetic activity caused by depression, worry and lassitude can induce intense gastrointestinal activity. Endocrine glands are also influenced by psychosomatic effects: the sympathetics (thalamus) controlling the adrenals, and the parasympathetics (hypothalamus) controlling the pituitary. The latter's response can be to produce several major hormones, including those which control metabolism.

Extreme nervous tension or anxiety—a psychosomatic effect—can be directly related to gastrointestinal disturbance. The typical psoriatic might or might not be a highly-strung, emotional individual. Nevertheless it is highly likely in many instances that psychological influences trigger a physiological chain reaction.

In this respect, to suggest that a disease is incurable, or to proclaim a state of ill-health as being terminal and subject to a time limit, is to assume an enormous responsibility for pronouncing a sentence upon the sufferer.

Psoriatic triggers

Given an inherited predisposition, it seems that at any age foods, vaccinations, infections, medications (including oral steroids and intra-muscular injections) and even injury to the skin can stimulate psoriasis when we carry the gene.

Another trigger, if indeed one needs to be found, is the state of mind. Equally, emotion and stress can be marked as triggers (some experts hold that psoriatics' emotional state results from their having psoriasis on their skin, while others dismiss altogether the suggestion that stress can produce a diseased state at all).

If stressed and emotional states set off an outbreak of psoriasis (as most people who suffer from it will assert is a plain and straightforward fact), then internal digestive, metabolic and endocrinal irregularities are the precipitating physiological agents that produce the symptoms evident on the skin. Furthermore, the physiological response can be symptomatic of an imbalance that occurs following an immune system reaction, or of the presence of yeast bacteria in the gut, and metabolic confusion at the very least.

'Trigger-happy' foods

Foods that can stimulate the incidence of psoriasis in some people who are indisposed to the disease include chocolate, caffeine, alcohol, mushrooms, peanuts, aubergine (eggplant), potatoes, tomatoes and bell peppers (capsicum). The last four foods are members of the nightshade family of plants, the *Solanaceae*. This family includes the just-listed aubergine, potatoes (but not sweet potatoes), tomatoes and bell peppers (in all colours), as well as paprika, chilli peppers, tobacco and Cape gooseberry.[25]

The nightshade family and alkaloids

The poisonous components (alkaloids) of some plants are used for medicinal purposes. Alkaloids are a large group of potent, nitrogen-containing alkaline substances. The plant deadly nightshade (*Solanum nigrum*) contains a deadly quantity of the alkaloids which in other plants, such as the potato, measures a mere 1 per cent of the plant's weight. The alkaloid solanine is obvious in the green potato (the result of exposure to light of an unripened potato), and makes it a danger to consume. The alkaloid piperidine in pepper irritates both digestive and urinary tracts. Caffeine in tea and coffee is another common form of alkaloid.

Most alkaloids have a bitter taste. As they are insoluble in water, the medicines in which alkaloids are used are provided in the form of tinctures (alcoholic solutions) and tablets. They can be extremely poisonous if accurate dosages are not adhered to. Alkaloids are also found in atropine (from the belladonna plant, *Atropa belladonna*), cocaine, morphine, codeine and other drugs derived from opium, nicotine, quinine and quinidine from Peruvian bark; and strychnine.

Paradoxically, psoriasis may be alleviated by other substances of the alkaloid 'family', including allantoin and berberine (see *Part III: Taking Control*, page 125).

Gluten

Gluten is present in the endosperm of grains and produces in some people a definite allergic reaction (coeliac disease). After milk, gluten represents the most common offender amongst food intolerance or allergy responses. Gluten is 78 per cent of the total protein in wheat and is a powerful intestinal irritant in those who are susceptible to its effects through its constituent gliadin.

Monosodium glutamate (MSG) is prepared commercially from gluten. Gluten is also present in stock cubes, canned soups, beer and any processed food that contains hydrolysed vegetable protein. MSG (additive code number 621) is widely used. Look for it in soy sauce, camembert, parmesan and blue vein cheeses, tomato paste, wine, and corn chips. MSG and hydrolysed vegetable protein are both dangerous excitotoxins.[26]

Stress

Remarkably, some trained professionals still decry the likelihood of stress being a factor in disease altogether, let alone in psoriasis flare-ups. Factually speaking, stress will cause significant physiological reactions, as will emotional upsets, distress and depression. Under extreme stress, the body reacts in the following ways:

- Capillaries connecting to muscles dilate to enable a greater passage of blood;
- Capillaries which are supplying organs that are non-essential to physical action close;
- Digestion ceases altogether;
- Hormones stimulate the heart to increase its rate and output, thereby increasing blood pressure and respiratory rate;
- Fats and sugars are released into the bloodstream, as fuel for the muscles;
- Cholesterol levels are raised; and
- Changes to the composition of the blood prepare the circulatory system for rapid clotting in case of injury.

If even certain low-level emotions can have an effect on the body's circulation, what happens when we boil over with anger? Dr Andrew Bell, MB, BS, MRCP, in *Creative Health*, cites the claim that the killing power of white blood cells is diminished. Conversely, the immune system is strengthened when a long-held secret is liberated.[27]

Our physiological response to modern day circumstances is really no different from our primitive ancestors' reaction to danger or life-threatening incidents. The main difference is that in our case physical reaction is usually not called for, with the following results:

- The ability to respond becomes depleted through lack of a physical comeback, which results in a distressed and over-stressed state;
- The thymus gland is shrunken and defective in its immune system control function, and consequently the vital lymphocytes are rendered powerless;
- Blood viscosity is maintained at a high level and blood flow is sluggish;
- Oxygen supply to body tissues is deprived; and
- General immunity-depletion results in lesser defence against harmful pathogens.

A psoriatic who is under stress has an automatic susceptibility to these vital factors which are typically already in decline, given the relationship to the disease of immune function, quality of blood supply, dehydration, oxygenation, indisposition towards fats and sugars in the blood supply, and already abnormal blood cholesterol levels.

The body can also experience physiological stress from high noise levels and lack of exercise and oxygen.

Arthritis and psoriasis

Psoriatics have a disposition towards developing arthritis later in life. Psoriasis underneath the fingernails or toenails in particular can have an interrelationship with arthritic psoriasis. Some form of arthritis is evident in 5 per cent of psoriasis sufferers and the same percentage of arthritis sufferers has some form of psoriasis. It is an alarming circumstance, considering the powers of modern medicine, that by the age of 60 nine out of ten people are victims of rheumatoid arthritis or osteoarthritis.[28] Rheumatoid arthritis is an autoimmune disease in which the cartilage which connects bone joints is attacked by the immune system.

While there are many factors inherent in the onset of arthritis—poor lubrication of the joints, allergies, hormonal imbalance, bone strain and deformities being amongst them—consider also the basic roles of diet and nutrition. Nutritionists recommend the avoidance of too much sugar, excitotoxins and other stimulants, and too much fat and protein. Levels of the amino acid cystine are much lower in arthritic patients. Cystine is a sulphur-containing amino acid that is reliant upon the presence of methionine; sulphur is used in ointments and creams to treat dermatitis, eczema and psoriasis.

Food production and processing

Further complications in achieving appropriate nutritional value from food arise when we consider the effects of production and processing methods on formerly fresh, vital food. It is generally known that the nutritive value present in many field-grown foods has decreased over recent decades, due to the depletion of soils and even the sterilisation of farming land by increasing reliance upon fertilisers, herbicides and pesticides, and largely indefensible monocultural farming practices.[29] Worldwide, we dump 100,000 per cent more chemicals on our precious farming lands today than were there at the end of World War II. Each of us who eats the common consumer foods will ingest another gallon of pesticides this year.[30] These poisons are stored in our tissues and organs.

Nutritive value is further eroded by food processing, the application of high heat levels, overcooking, pasteurisation and the insurgence of additives and non-natural preservatives to prolong shelf-life and improve the appearance of products. In addition, the residue of toxins from pesticide and herbicide treatments used in the growing process can do nothing for the body that is striving to make the most of the fuel with which it is supplied. Our production methods are too clever for our own good and sometimes border on the absurd. For example, quite apart from the questionable practice of battery-farming in the commercial poultry and egg industries, in the stipulated 'quality control' processes the porous egg shells are treated with mineral oil to replace the natural protective oil which was removed during the washing process. Virtually every 'fresh' (non-organically grown) food we select from the shelves has been tampered with in some way.

Hydrogenation, which was originally developed for the soap industry, is a process used in food production to render fat substances free of rancidity and organic decay. Since its introduction to, and subsequent revolution of, the food industry in the years following World War II, hydrogenation has been joined by a veritable onslaught of clever applications of chemistry to address the commercial requirements of food processing, storage and shelf-life. Brilliant chemists have also been put to work to develop colour, flavour and visual enhancers for foods, very many of which end up being little more than poisons disguised as food. Hence what once were fine providers of nutrition have become vehicles for benzoates, nitrites, nitrates, propionates and sorbates. Numerous works have been published to warn consumers about the dangers of these products. Conversely, food-processing apologists proclaim its advantages as having made the world safer and improved diets. If we accept that 'fresh is best', suffice to say that if food is processed, contains refined sugar or refined flour, or has been in any way deranged by the presence of artificially induced 'enhancements' or non-natural preservatives, it does not in any way meet the definition of food, that is, 'material which nourishes'.

It is not only for the benefit of the allergy-prone that food labelling (the requirement to list ingredients on the container's label) is necessary. It is essential for all consumers. We have a fundamental right to know what we are going to ingest. Australians have led the world in convincing our government that we have the right to know when foods have been genetically modified. We are not so lucky when it comes to food irradiation. Both have moral implications. Even before these 'improvements' were foisted upon us, we have for decades the world over been ingesting substances in processed foods and water supplies which are known to have serious and harmful consequences for the human animal. These toxins are cumulative. This further supports the already strong case for the avoidance of processed and refined foods in the diet. The presence of psoriasis and the susceptibility of our digestive, metabolic and autoimmune systems cries out for a careful and kindly attention to detail in evaluating everything that is loaded into the body. (See also *Table 1* in *Appendix 1*.)

Additives and excitotoxins

Excititoxins are for the most part acidic amino acids which react with brain receptors in a way that promotes the destruction of certain types of neurons. In this respect they are classed as neurotoxins. Some of them are capable of penetrating the blood–brain barrier, contrary to their manufacturers' claims.[31] Monosodium glutamate, for example, penetrates the barrier. Since so many foods in the common consumer's diet are laced with MSG, this neurotoxin thus has direct access to, and is niggling away at, the brain on a regular basis.

Perhaps the most alarming of these dangerous insurgents—amongst the long list of food additives which are known to be highly toxic and hazardous, and which food licensing authorities such as the US Food and Drug Administration (FDA) and the Australia New Zealand Food Authority (ANZFA) have approved as safe 'foods'—is aspartame (additive code number 951). This artificial sweetener is implicated in several neurodegenerative diseases. The methyl ester in aspartame becomes methanol (wood alcohol). When exposed to temperatures above 86°F (28°C), methanol converts to formaldehyde and then to formic acid. Some research shows that methanol toxicity imitates multiple sclerosis.[32] Formaldehyde crosses the blood–brain barrier to wreak havoc on neurotransmitter function.

A 30-page document presented in the early 1980s by the US National Soft Drinks Association warned of the dangers of aspartame, yet the FDA approved its use in foods and in soft drinks. In that decade it was established that aspartame could affect brain chemistry—it inhibited the synthesis of neurotransmitters such as serotonin. In 1985, 400,000 tons of aspartame were consumed in the United States alone. It was expected that by late 2000, one billion pounds (200 million kilograms) of aspartame would be consumed.[33] Documented symptoms of aspartame disease range from coma to death.[34] Aspartame is used in more than 90 countries as an additive in breakfast cereals, sweets, desserts, lollies, soft drinks, tea beverages, instant coffees, cola and cocoa drinks, sugar-free gum and mints, juice drinks, flavoured milk drinks, health supplements, yoghurts, to name but a few.

Incomprehensibly, excitotoxins of one form or another are added to an incredibly long list of processed foods. They can be identified in soy protein extract, flavourings, spices and yeast extracts. Their presence in liquid forms in soups, sauces and drinks presents even greater dangers than in solid foods, because of their more ready availability for absorption. Are we being deliberately poisoned here?

Aspartame is one of seven artificial sweeteners approved for use in Australia, along with saccharin, acelphame K and cyclamate. These products are marketed as alternatives to sugar and therefore as a 'non-fattening diet aid'. Ironically, according to a study published in the British medical journal *The Lancet*, aspartame has the effect of increasing the appetite and particularly the desire for carbohydrates, known 'fatteners'.[35] Furthermore, by turning to diet potato crisps to satisfy this craving, diet drink faddists can lay themselves open to the food additive olestra. This 'fake fat' is approved (by the FDA) as an additive to some brands of 'light' potato crisps—despite its ability to incite 'gastric irritation and anal leakage', according to the health warning on the packaging.

The effects of excititoxins are long-term, subtle and insinuating, their use a violation of the fundamental right to good health and well-being.

Static

The human nervous system is susceptible to the energy fields of external elements. Yet we are caught in the deepest recesses of a severe electromagnetic storm, which is intensifying. Just as the demand for convenience has fuelled the proliferation of easy-to-deal-with 'food' products, our need for instant communication, entertainment and information storage and exchange has propelled us headlong into an energy crisis. The problem of electromagnetic exposure is not only caused by the most obvious—microwave radiation, mobile phones and high-voltage power lines. In a 1982 edition of *The Lancet*, it was noted that exposure to office fluorescent lighting was implicated in a 2½ times increase in the risk of melanomas.[36] The incidence of cancer has risen from one in nine people in 1900 to one in two people at 2000. At this rate, we can all get it if we so desire.

Psoriasis is neither caused by nor, as far as we yet know, triggered by electromagnetic fields. However, in consideration of the general health picture which underlies the condition, it pays to be aware of all hazards to daily living.

The future

Modern medicine is peopled by some brilliant individuals and has been successful in ridding human existence of some 'old' diseases. However, almost as soon as these are eradicated, new pathogens are identified, as if it is a natural requirement of a normal life pattern to be restrained and controlled by disease. In many instances, the newly identified diseases are mutations of the older forms, and are therefore resistant to the 'cure'. Many such diseases are caused by pathogens or parasites which are successful in using the body's normal processes to protect themselves against the body's natural immune system response. They develop a protective cloak of proteins, which fools the immune system into thinking that the parasite is actually a part of normal body structure and behaviour, a so-called self cell. Thus, when neutrophils encounter the protected parasite, they do not recognise the invader and it is left alone to proliferate.[37]

If allopathic, molecular medicine cannot keep pace with the epidemics of disease and rampant physiological degeneration with which the world is faced, let alone the proliferation of new mutations, if drug therapy is not the answer, and if governments and regulatory authorities are on the one hand not infallible and on the other impotent against business—some of which apparently is too big to be bothered by conscience—where does the answer lie?

PART II

Diary of a psoriatic

I am elated because I have the power to reverse a serious bout
of psoriasis. I also can control it whenever I lapse in my self-
treatment. I do not allow psoriasis to bother me; there are many
ways to live with it and control it. Glibly, I wrote in some notes
in the mid-1980s, 'If I want to have psoriasis,
I know how to go about getting it.'
Today I enjoy a 99 per cent remission 99 per cent of the time.

4 How I overcame psoriasis and learned to live with it

A personal profile

As an introduction to a personal story and in the genuine spirit of the exercise, here is a personal profile (albeit superficial, coming as it does from my own hand): I am regarded as a naturally outgoing person, creative and with a liberal sense of humour that is bent far left of reverent and often a touch too obscure for some people. As an extrovert rather than introvert, I am less likely to approach something in a calm and moderate manner, leaning more towards the dramatic and overt (hence I wear a disease rather than internalise it). I have worked in jobs that require a certain degree of extroversion, and the ability to develop and maintain the respect and commitment of others who have very healthy egos and are assertive to at least the same degree. Specifically, I have worked as a writer and producer in media, advertising and the recording industry and for the past ten years have produced clients' résumés and job applications. I have also acted in the studio and on stage; so how I look has been very important to me from time to time, and therefore I also possess a sense of pride.

I am a Leo, although not a typical one in that I am not into 'gold or jewellery', and a Rabbit in Chinese astrology. My tastes are fairly refined; I really enjoy good wine and prefer tasty (sometimes rich) foods over bland foods. I have vacillated between a 'sweet tooth' and preferences for the savoury. As an ectomorph, my weight is right for my height. My complexion is dark with an olive, oily skin which tans easily, and I am hirsute (bearded, thick long hair).

I am equally happy ensconced before the hi-fi with Frank Zappa enlightening the household, swimming at the beach or mucking about in the garden. Overall, I prefer to avoid crowds and at a party will opt for conversation in a corner over dancing on the tables. I inherited green thumbs (albeit psoriatic—there is no psoriasis in either parent), and have had several organic and biodynamic vegetable and herb gardens. Often gardening, with casual walks, has represented the sum of my exercise pattern and as strenuous exercise and sport are not for me (I have not even the slightest interest in watching it). The work I do makes for a rather sedentary lifestyle and I am formulating the firm decision to adopt a daily commitment to stretches, if only to help delay the onset of arthritic stiffness.

While I was extremely successful with self-hypnosis, I have never been able to achieve the meditative state—neither by sitting cross-legged nor contemplating a bean. Nevertheless, I have experienced deep levels of consciousness by other methods, and have what I believe is a reasonable cosmology. From time to time metaphysics has presented very great interest. With my first readings in this at age fifteen, a fair assessment has evolved, and I am always reviewing my beliefs.

An idealist and a perfectionist, I apparently expect the same in others and am not mad about people who are content with mediocrity, either their own or that of anyone or anything. There can be a fairly short fuse on this side of temper. While I try to follow natural laws, spiritual tranquillity can elude me because of arrogance and rigidity in my thinking sometimes. I am not the best companion with whom to watch the evening news.

I believe that the human mind and soul—distinct and separate from each other, though connected by their common foundation—possess fragments of the source of all life, whatever it might be and by whatever name you want it to go by. This source must be infinitely more intelligent than everything else. Therefore you and I possess a spark which must be the most sacred thing we know. We do not need priests, professors or channelled entities to inform us of it or describe it for us, to save us from ourselves, or to lead us to any promised land. While it might be true that self-styled 'gurus' stimulate our search and enlightenment (if that is what we seek), and in so doing cause us to instigate some worthwhile changes for ourselves, they can only lead us to the promised land that *they* know—which is automatically corrupted by virtue of their act of wishing to lead and influence us. ('He who claims to teach is really receiving a lesson', to paraphrase J. Krishnamurti.)[1] Higher consciousness is attainable without withdrawing to a mountain cave or desert dugout; it is omnipresent even on the 44th floor of an office block. Ultimately we will do it ourselves, for we possess the impulse, the understanding and the access. Perhaps this is the real message of the 'Age of Aquarius', the time in our long history when we can shuck off the shackles of conditioning and manipulation, as true individuals with a common origin and a shared destiny.

(Having read the draft, my wife, Deborah pencilled at the bottom of the page, *I am a certified megalomaniac performance artist*, so that pretty well completes the picture.)

Since 1982

It is the Australian summer of 2000–2001. Since 1981, I have experienced two periods of quite bad psoriatic 'attacks'. These coincided with my disregard for some of the basic dietary rules laid down elsewhere in this book and which I formulated as the result of research that began in 1980. The most severe relapses also occurred at the times I was under stress related to my working life or milieu—in the late 1980s—early 1990s when I was in a job that was frustrating and lacking in creative satisfaction and professional esteem, and in the late 1990s when I was going through a period of similar dissatisfaction with my daily lot, and wanting to pursue 'serious' writing. The earlier period was quite long-lasting, and was also characterised by economic uncertainty and worries about being able to make ends meet each week. My wife recalls having to vacuum the living room floor each morning, because my distracted scratching each evening created piles of white scale on the rug. She jokes of also having to vacuum the bed sheets each day. I had psoriasis quite badly on my legs and torso, nearly always on my scalp, and on the elbows. The embarrassment caused by this condition meant that I spent the whole of several summers in a very hot and humid atmosphere, always dressed in long pants, where I would otherwise have opted for shorts.

'Cow cream'

In the early 1990s I was alerted to a discovery made by a member of the Australian Psoriasis Association, of a cream which veterinarians used to lubricate and heal cows' teats. This person, who at the time suffered with psoriasis on her hands and fingers, found that her lesions abated in severity after she applied the cream to her cows' teats. The cream is sold in Australia as a proprietary veterinary ointment. Its active constituents are zinc oxide, which is used in many skin treatments, and boric (or boracic) acid, a mild antiseptic. Judging by its mild smell, these are presented in a lanolin (wool fat) base. Its label attests to its use 'to assist in the healing of cracks, sores and wounds' and 'to prevent chapping and infections on cows' teats and udders'. The ointment was made available through the Australian Psoriasis Association, with a caution to discontinue its use if irritations occurred. This was indeed the case in my experience with it, on some occasions, when small pimple-like eruptions would appear on the patches that were treated. I still have the remains of a one-pound (500 g) jar (A\$20.30 from a local vet in 1998).

So yes, I used the 'cow cream', as I have long called it, for many years. I must admit this is the result of a rather mindless preoccupation with convenience. Had I been true to myself all this time, I would have been using natural cold-pressed seed oils or any of the other oils I wrote about 20 years ago. Nevertheless, the 'cow cream' was highly effective in removing the hard dry white scale. Secondly, it served as a convenient barrier to the municipal water supply—I used to apply it to the spots, variously many and few as they were during those years, before the morning's shower. One of this cream's greatest drawbacks is its greasiness, which can discolour and ruin garments. Considering the nature of this treatment and the many years I used it, it is ironic—and not a little disappointing—that I had considerably less success with a specifically dedicated and considerably more expensive natural treatment, as described below.

Fingernails and toenails

Throughout the period 1988–99, I suffered a lot with pustular psoriasis— blistering and badly cracked fingers, especially the fingertips and the undersides and sides of the fingers, never on the palm or top of the fingers or hands. This was accompanied by extensive psoriasis under my fingernails and toenails. It is a particularly distressing form for people whose hands are in front of clients each day, for those who work with tools and in cold conditions, or those whose hands are in water and in contact with foreign materials. The warping of my big toenails caused by the crust beneath them has permanently changed the shape of a pair of deck shoes. It also necessitated trimming and filing my toenails twice a week, because their distorted shapes made it painful to wear shoes. The nails also tore holes in socks. The dead skin cells that accumulate beneath the nail can develop a particularly awful aroma, too, and the general appearance is discolouration, yellowed usually, and the nail itself can be quite brittle.

The blistering and cracked fingers were an especially awful experience, as this meant open wounds that were highly susceptible to being harmed and did not enjoy being in water. The rough, peeling skin also caught on clothing fibres.

For many of these years I wore disposable latex gloves when showering, and even when working in the garden. One evening, Deborah and I were to help out at a Scout fund-raising event. I was to work behind the bar. I was so embarrassed by the state of my hands that Deb suggested I wear white gloves. She had to shop around to find the appropriate kind of cotton gloves. So I wouldn't look like a complete dork, I carried the effect through to full 'fancy dress', with bow tie and wing collar. Deb dressed in a similarly formal fashion, complete with white gloves, to help me get away with the ruse.

There was a definite abatement of symptoms any time I was out of town. I attributed this improvement to lack of contact with the municipal water supply and at home avoided all possible contact directly to my hands.

Water

I love to drink water and have no problem with taking the recommended eight large glasses a day. For many years our family bought spring water. While we have been fortunate to live in a city where the water supply is not fluoridated, nevertheless the tap water invariably smells like a swimming pool, such is its level of chlorination. Of course, chlorine is only one of numerous chemicals that are added to the average municipal water supply (the majority are colourless, odourless and tasteless). So for years we had bulk supplies of spring water delivered weekly and used this exclusively for cooking and drinking. In more recent times, we have added a rainwater catchment and filtering system, and enjoy delicious, energising water that is as pure as it can be expected in an inner-city area.

Water therapy

I was for a time interested in an alternative water therapy, namely urine therapy. An Australian author, Harald W. Tietze, has written much on this subject, which I first became aware of in the 1970s. Ever since coming upon the knowledge, I had applied my urine to gain immediate relief from bites from large black 'sugar' ants, and believed strongly enough in the stories I had heard to be prepared to take my own urine should I be the victim of a snakebite. (Valuable, apparently, because of the body producing its own antivenene; this is so far personally untried!). Urine is sterile; it is also antibacterial and antifungal. It has been used for centuries as an effective healing agent and its by-product, urea, is used in many skin creams and beauty treatments. The first time I had the courage to ingest it occurred quite spontaneously during a 'sojourn in the wilderness', which is touched on below.

Much later, in 1998, when I was really suffering with the discomfort and unwieldiness of pustular psoriasis, I spent a couple of weeks religiously following the directions in Mr Tietze's handbook *Water Medicine*. In my first encounter, I had taken the urine orally. Following Mr Tietze's directions, I began each day with topical dabs of urine collected mid-stream from the first passing of the day, and which I stored for a few days. I have to admit that I discontinued this therapy because of the odour. I couldn't get away from it; even though the program preceded the daily shower and shampoo the odour seemed to be ingrained in my pores.

You might assume from this that I am willing to try anything in the pursuit of relief from psoriasis. Not quite. In juxtaposition, I would like you to consider whether you would be prepared to try urine therapy, in the light of your unlikely use at some time of any one of the orthodox treatments such as corticosteroids which you know can cause great harm to your body?

Climate and lifestyle

Since 1988 I have lived in a hot, humid, subtropical city close to the coast and within an hour's drive of some fabulous beaches with their attendant therapeutic salt water and sunshine. When I published *Sor-i-a-sis* I was living on the Australian east coast and swam regularly. Between 1982 and 1984, and again between 1986 and 1988, I lived in tableland regions and therefore more temperate climes. Winters were fierce, with light snow on a couple of occasions and severe frosts, and summer days were warm, often dry.

For most of this period I had a fabulous job as a writer and producer with a commercial radio station, worked long hours and, as a period of temporary 'bachelorhood' coincided with this time, participated in events and functions that meant lots of alcohol, and some very odd meal times. Pizza and take-away roast chicken figured largely, as did buckets of (instant) coffee at all times of day and night. I smoked heavily, too. Psoriasis was ever-present.

Between 1984 and 1986, I lived on the coast again and swam and surfed through winter, but worked in a similar role with the attendant lifestyle.

Hyperthyroidism

During 1992–93, I was diagnosed with hyperthyroidism, discovered quite by chance by a diligent general practitioner whom I had consulted about a severe influenza. He thought that my eyes were slightly bulging, a tell-tale symptom, and arranged for the necessary pathology tests. Hyperthyroidism was confirmed, and I duly set off on a course of consultations with an endocrinologist who treated me with carbimazole. I was really the last person to accept a future dependent upon a treatment such as this (the hormone inhibits the production of iodine, which in the hyperthyroid condition is over-produced by an over-enthusiastic thyroid gland), so I was greatly relieved when, approximately eighteen months later, tests confirmed that everything had returned to normal.

Hyperthyroidism can arise through the effect on the endocrine system induced by the hypothalamus stimulating the thyroid gland into secreting the excess thyroid hormone that underlies the condition. I was quite overweight during this period and generally exhibited a fairly sluggish constitution and lethargy.

Testing new products

Between 1996 and 1997 I endured another period of road-testing some new products. This became an endurance because of the overall ineffectiveness of the products in my particular circumstances. It was also a matter of bad timing on my part and failure to realise that there was something else affecting me then.

I discontinued the treatments—having used soap, shampoo, conditioner, morning and evening skin lotions, and black mud packs—when spots on my legs became quite irritated by the skin lotion, coinciding with a 30 per cent price rise in the shampoo. From the time I made the initial purchase until I abandoned the treatments eight months later, I used all the products. Some temporary and rapid reduction in the severity of the spots on my legs followed use of the mud pack, but generally speaking I was not the right person for these products at that time. (While writing these pages, I retrieved the remaining tube of nourishing cream from the original batch and gave it another run, but it soon incited inflammation.) This is a different experience from the incidence of a 'healing crisis' known in naturopathy and homeopathy, where a condition will worsen temporarily during its progress to remission.

A change of routine

Christmas and New Year 1998–99 saw me enjoying a couple of weeks in the sun and surf and away from the offending water supply, using very little in the way of surface treatments and enjoying a varied diet which included not only fresh foods and juices but also 'bacon and eggs', coffee, glutenous bread and alcohol. I was totally clear. I was especially relieved to be rid of the cracked and blistering fingers. These symptoms, together with guttate spots on my torso and legs, returned soon after the holiday was over and I had returned to my daily routine.

Cheese!

In 1999, I made an awesome discovery—more a rediscovery, really, as the key was in that original slim volume *Sor-i-a-sis*. It totally turned my life around. Since the 1970s, I had eaten a lot of dairy products even though I knew from my research that one should avoid them, at least in the earliest and mid-stages of treating psoriasis. When I say I ate a lot of dairy products, I mean not so much the quantity as the frequency. During the late seventies I bought raw fresh milk from farms nearby, and made cottage cheese and yoghurt. This was a very enjoyable pastime: the cheeses hung outdoors and the whey (which regulates the secretion of gastric acid, incidentally) was collected and used for its lactic acid (in bread mixes and on muesli). Natural lactic acid stimulates the pancreas. Neither the cheese nor the yoghurt was very good for the psoriatic, however, and photographs from this time clearly show thick white crusts on my knees, shins and elbows. It hadn't occurred to me at this stage to apply anything to remove these crusts.

For about ten years (mid-eighties to mid-nineties), most mornings I would eat a combination of yoghurt, stewed rhubarb and tahini; sometimes fresh watermelon or pawpaw and yoghurt. In more recent years I have had a lot of enjoyment from cheese and crackers, preferring the vintaged and richer styles—aged cheddar, sometimes blue cheese, often camembert and brie. Cheddar is very high in saturated fats; blue vein and Stilton (which also contain about 35 per cent fat) contain amines and MSG.

Coffee

Meanwhile I had stopped drinking coffee in, let's say, 1994. When I say coffee, I mean *coffee*! I like it fresh, strong and black. Up until about 1992, I used to have cream with it and insisted on freshly brewed espresso, never instant, and was indignant of failure to produce a strong, flavour-filled cup. Now here is where it gets rather personal. For about eight years, I had suffered from what I thought was haemorrhoids. I don't have to describe the sensation or the physical nature of this ailment. Well, sometimes I 'had them' really badly. It was this experience that made me quit my beloved coffee. I learned around this time that tea and coffee shared alkaloids that could have similarly adverse effects on the psoriatic. So I was pretty much off both.

I still drank wine, however; I ate cheese, yoghurt, and other trigger foods such as capsicum, eggplant and chocolate. Capsicum was a favourite ingredient in many a meal, as was tomato, and I used to like an open sandwich of tomato and peanut butter. (To be told that capsicum, eggplant and wine were out was really amongst the most boring and unwelcome news I had ever heard.) I ate ice cream, and a nosh of prawns, oysters and crab was simultaneous with the beach experience.

A new upsurge: eczema or pruritus ani?

My excruciating problem persisted. My skin—the psoriatic one—suffered a serious upsurge in 1997–98. I was faced with the real threat of a major torso coverage and my fingers and hands were cracked and blistering, a hideous experience. During a weekend at the beach I had noticed an immediate improvement—a relaxation, if you like, of the intense stress in my fingers. I had attributed this to the change in water supply and remained with this assumption for many months.

My problems persisted, and in the interim a GP mentioned a form of eczema of the anus (EOTA). This cropped up again when researching the permeable intestine factor and in particular the incidence of a diseased pancreas. I must admit I didn't do any research into this personally. At the time I was really having problems; I was suffering in my own shadow and really could not get interested in the subject. I'm sure a lot of readers can identify with this feeling; it's probably common amongst us psoriatics at one time or another.

The condition still crops up from time to time, although never as severely or as prolonged as then, and I can usually pinpoint the reason—one or another exacerbating substance in the diet. This excruciating condition shares many characteristics with pruritus ani, a fairly common form of contact dermatitis. Basically, one grows troublesome bacteria in one's bum! The growth of germs and fungi is promoted by the productive sweat glands and the warm and moist conditions which are present in the 'normal' anal area.

My problem was at its worst during a very hot and humid summer, when my work entailed being seated on a chair, usually in front of a word processor. My underwear was cotton (non-synthetic, so it breathed), the chair was leather. After much trial and experimentation, the most immediate and longest-lasting relief was obtained from a simple papaya ointment (and usually only one application was necessary). Deficiencies of vitamin A, B complex and iron are implicated in the rectal skin disorder. *Skin Troubles* (from Science of Life Books) gives advice on the use of vitamin E taken in a dosage of 400–600mg daily.[2]

All along I knew that there were dietary–digestive factors at work here, and that corrections to some important dietary habits were all that were needed to be comfortable. While it really is as simple as this, it isn't always easy, is it?

The point is, I knew what was happening and I didn't do much about it. Sometimes it is so easy to keep on doing what we do, and so hard to make a change—to accept a state of suffering and not respond practically with what we know instinctively or have learned.

Animal by-products

We can never be certain that foods we consume do not contain some animal by-product. I turned to partial-vegetarianism in 1977 but still eat and enjoy seafood, organic chicken, eggs and butter. If I eat meat from sheep, cows or pigs, I suffer an adverse reaction. This first was evident to me in 1984. I was at a friend's barbecue, and the aroma of sizzling lamb shashlik was just too much for me. As a meat eater, I used to revel in rare char-grilled steaks, and to this day ancient genes send my tastebuds soaring on the promising smell of roasting meat. This night, however, I made an amazing discovery. I couldn't resist some barbecued lamb. Within a couple of hours my legs and trunk erupted in red weals that itched and burned with a deep irritation which could not be relieved by scratching or rubbing. The attack lasted several hours.

I have experienced the same sensation on several occasions over the years, after succumbing to a similar loss of self-control in the presence of sizzling bacon, say, or a particularly fine leg ham at the Christmas table. Sometimes it occurs inadvertently. The importance of this reaction is that I know immediately when a food I have eaten contains animal by-products. For example, several years ago, my wife and I were at the State Art Gallery and interrupted our meanderings with a bite to eat in the bistro. I ordered the 'vegetarian' pie, and as has been my wont since the shashlik experience, had the waitress confirm that it indeed was 'vegetarian'. However, less than an hour later I felt the familiar burning and itching in several spots on my legs. I assumed that there must have been some beef shortening in the pastry crust. So you can never be really certain, can you?

You might be interested to know that pig fat is used in some ice creams, particularly the soft twirly types. Even so-called 'natural' ice creams, priced at the top of the range, cause the same eruptions on my skin. With the benefit of hindsight afforded by the research for this book, I recognise here the link with the body's production of eosinophils in response to an inability to metabolise the proteins in cow's milk or animal meats (as described in *Leaky Gut Syndrome* in *Part I*).

Coffee off the hook

In 1998, some friends returned from a holiday in Tasmania with a promised vintage cheddar from a producer renowned for fine quality cheeses. It was a fabulously sharp block, so sharp in fact that others with whom we shared it returned their portions. I relished it, and when Deb and I joined some other friends for a holiday at South West Rocks in New South Wales, we took the last of the block to share.

Now, I was really looking forward to this holiday. I worked hard at a job that was intense and demanding, so there was no way I was going to have it marred by EOTA! I spent the whole week shying away from coffee and working around capsicum, tomatoes, eggplant et al. Nightly we enjoyed the delicious vintage cheddar with some mighty wines. Daily I bled and squirmed.

At home again, I thought back over the week and tried to work out what could have caused such suffering. It's easy to say, with hindsight, that the culprit was plain to see, but it was not so at the time. I eventually deduced that it must have been the cheese, so I avoided it in all forms for two weeks. EOTA vanished! Right, I thought, let's try the old coffee. So for two weeks I drank coffee every day, without any (EOTA) side-effects. The program called next for two weeks of cheese and coffee. I lasted only a day or so on the combination, because as soon as the cheese hit my system it went straight to my anus armed with gasoline and razorblades!

This was a monumental discovery. To this day, I drink and enjoy coffee the way I have always liked it—I went without it for nearly five years!—but if I sneak so much as a nibble of cheese in the dark of night, I pay for it next morning. It simply isn't worth it. It also means forgoing parmesan cheese in one of my favourite dishes, pesto. Meanwhile, it's important to say that this is not an endorsement of coffee. Anyone who is serious about pursuing natural health would agree that coffee is not the ideal ally.

Changing tastes

Nevertheless, as I have found with any food item, once discarded and successfully avoided, my taste for it diminishes and ultimately vanishes. Nowadays, I can't abide the taste of yoghurt, and while I think I would love to have some cheese and crackers with a favourite wine in the afternoon light, the fatty dairy smell of cheese turns me off. I find ice cream passé, and overall am frightened off almost all dairy products by the recollection of my sufferings with EOTA. I still prefer butter over margarine (because it's a matter of natural versus synthetic), and like the effect of cold hard butter on crunchy toast. Some habits never die, it seems. In the end, however, any habit is worth committing to the recycle bin if it's anathema to our system. Once again, our body—our skin—is the finest litmus test of what is right and what is not right for us. We are each an individual, but some things we have in common.

Osteopathy and Rolfing

The year 1999 was marked by a chronic condition of another kind— excruciating pain in my neck and shoulders that proved remarkably intractable. It was the result of protracted periods at the word processor, and largely attributable to the placement of my work-station in a new office and to the way I positioned myself before it. I spent eight to ten hours each day there. There was another, esoteric factor in this, namely pent-up tension, or frustrated creativity, with impending creative energy welling and awaiting release (such as writing this book has afforded).

Regular visits to an osteopath for five weeks and a series of stretches and exercises were of considerable benefit. I decided to augment this treatment with a further course of treatment intended to correct my posture. For this I thought the Alexander technique, Feldenkrais or the Rolf method would suffice. The latter won when Deborah noticed an advertisement for a structural integration practitioner in the community newspaper. When I told my osteopath of the decision to pursue rolfing he remarked, 'You're about to discover a whole new meaning of pain!'

The structural integration practitioner was excellent and we struck a fine rapport. This is essential considering the levels of pain which accompany the extremely deep tissue massage and the intimacy of the treatment. Essentially, this system, developed by Dr Ida P. Rolf, lengthens and opens the patterns in the connective tissue (collagen). This then becomes softer and more pliable, and greatly improves flexibility and movement. 'Before' and 'after' photographs clearly demonstrate the corrections to the body's alignment following the ten sessions. I gained height, corrected a definite twist in my upper torso, the result of a serious car accident in 1971, and, perhaps most importantly, regained balance. While I would recommend the Rolf method of structural integration as a very beneficial treatment, it is not for everyone with a serious case of psoriasis, because there would be areas of the body that could not be treated, and the program would be incomplete. I was relieved of a lot of the pain and discomfort in my shoulders, but it did persist at a certain level.

Rolfing was temporarily interrupted in November by a holiday in Fiji.

While there, as a novice devotee of pain through deep tissue massage, I underwent a session with a Fijian who deserves renown for his talents for penetrating bare flesh with his fingers and thumbs. I have never known pain like it—it made my rolfer seem like a pussycat in comparison. This holiday is also mentioned for its relevance to diet and my experiences with skin problems afterwards. In Fiji virtually every meal included spicy food. This is not good for a psoriatic, even though at the time my skin was pretty clear— except for bits on my scalp and what by this time were chronic nail pits and plaque beneath toenails, thumbs and some fingernails. There was no psoriasis, nor had there been all year, on my elbows and knees.

The Fijian holiday was profoundly relaxing. I enjoyed the kava experience, and in this discovered a beneficial substance for intestinal health and sleeplessness. On return to Australia, I resumed the weekly rolfing sessions (with only one or two to go), and suddenly had to deal with a series of bizarre skin complaints. They were variously fungal in appearance, erythematic, and even during one manifestation bore a resemblance to molluscum contagiosum, reference to which is made below. There began a series of consultations with a brilliant and insightful Chinese practitioner who applies traditional therapies with orthodox training and qualifications. I was prescribed traditional herbal mixtures, natural creams, including vitamin A (retinol) cream, and even a steroid cream (hydrocortisone). I was warned off hot and spicy foods, and generally those foods and condiments which cause heat in the body. This is generally true of psoriatics. In the Chinese medical tradition, our affliction, being a 'red' disease, is not helped by overheating our constitution.

I totally stuffed up on one occasion, when I used tea-tree oil by self-administration, and caused myself a lot of drama and discomfort. This also sent me off on a second-guessing consultation with a totally orthodox GP. I am profoundly embarrassed by having placed myself in a situation that caused me to question the Chinese doctor—totally unnecessary considering my role in causing the problem. This orthodox consultation was nevertheless interesting, because it led to a discussion about psoriasis. 'Oh,' the doctor said, 'there's very little research done into psoriasis because the drug companies realise there would be no money in it for them.'

I completed the course of Chinese herbs, finished the rolfing series with great satisfaction, and overcame some strange new skin conditions. The cortisone cream lies unused in a bathroom cupboard.

Incidentally, the problem with my neck and shoulders persisted until one evening as I sat slumped in front of the television I sent my index finger and thumb on an exploratory mission to different points which the rolfing had alerted me to. I found automatic relief of my own accord, and on the few occasions the shoulder problem has resurfaced, I have been successful in gaining immediate relief.

How I overcame psoriasis

I was born in 1951. At the age of ten, when I was accustomed to wearing shorts as part of my school summer uniform, I became very embarrassed by two small red spots on my right thigh and shin which gradually became encrusted with a white scale and rapidly grew to three to four times their original diameter. My immediate reaction was to scratch the surface to remove the unsightly blotches which I was sure everyone was staring at. No sooner had I done this than a watery suppuration appeared, and a stinging soreness which made me wish I had left things alone. This was hard to do, of course.

Looking back, I recalled that this first experience with psoriasis was preceded by the sudden appearance of the not uncommon skin condition, molluscum contagiosum. This was diagnosed during the first few days of a summer holiday at the beach, when the blisters erupted on my lower legs. The condition often struck people who swam regularly in the public swimming pools, according to the dermatologists' directory of the day.[3] It was treated successfully. Shortly afterwards, however, I was struck down by tonsillitis. It was after this that psoriasis first appeared; presumably this was the trigger for which my psoriatic genes were waiting, although there had been plenty of similar opportunities previously.

Some years later, in 1965, I was herded, along with every other adolescent in the school, for the compulsory tuberculosis (TB) vaccination, a shot of streptomycin, an antibiotic which none of us needed. Streptomycin was first cultured from a soil mould in 1944 and developed in 1947; meanwhile TB had been largely removed from Western culture in 1945.[4] Amongst streptomycin's side-effects are skin rashes and fever. If any one of us who was vaccinated had been amongst the 3 per cent of the total world population unfortunate enough to get a dose of TB, a course of vitamin D to promote the production of some natural macrophages would probably have been sufficient remedy.

The city where I grew up is today an evolving habitat of the health renaissance, and can offer all of the varieties of popular orthomolecular therapies. In the dark conservative days of the early 1960s, however, consultation, diagnosis and, more often than not treatment, were relegated to the friendly chemist. So it was that my mother took me along to the pharmacist who admitted that he was not certain what had erupted on my leg, suggesting instead that the town's best dermatologist be consulted.

I recall that a brief visual examination was all that was required for this gentleman to diagnose psoriasis, which I initially had difficulty pronouncing. His prognosis was brief and to the point: I had an incurable skin disease about which the profession knew very little, much less its cause. With friendly professional bravado he offered his speciality, which was PUVA (ultraviolet light therapy—see page 119). We declined, and instead were given a prescription for an ointment. To the best of my memory, it afforded a period of remission. Nevertheless, having introduced itself, the affliction became more or less chronic, variously affecting my elbows, knees, scalp and both legs.

Belonging as we did to the culture of the time that never questioned orthodox treatments, let alone was aware of alternatives, my family and I sought no other possible courses of treatment. Instead we remained with the presumption that I suffered this 'incurable skin disease' which I would just have to learn to live with, all the while looking for and leaning on any new ointment or cream. Along with countless other sufferers and their families we became shareholders by proxy in the various drug companies.

Throughout my teens and even into my twenties and thirties, I had bad acne (which reduced in its severity as I gained years), which was no doubt attributable to hormonal activity, fairly intense emotional states and a taste for rich foods fuelled by the common apathy and ignorance of adolescence. At home, nutrition was middle-class Australian—this was in the days when health food stores specialised in cachoux and icing sugar, and a diet was about losing weight. Our diet was good, however—I ate hearty home-cooked meals with abundant fresh fruit and vegetables, and we drank rainwater collected in galvanised iron tanks at the side of the house. We even bathed in it for many years. I had acne as often as I had sweets, which was regularly.

Leaving home at sixteen, psoriasis and I lived in Sydney until 1977, where we made it to executive status as a 'company man' with a respected international manufacturer, and the attendant sacrifices of diet and lifestyle. Away from home there was less consideration for nutrition, as in the early days 'raging' meant getting drunk, and dining meant filling up with whatever was fancied, tasted good or was most readily available. In retrospect, it is easy to see in those years and in that lifestyle a gradual and inexorable toxification, the loading of the body and psyche with poisons of one kind or another as well as 'nourishment'—or at best setting up for or exacerbating a metabolic imbalance or enzyme derangement.

A road accident in 1971 caused me superficial though extensive head injuries. I cannot recall whether or not psoriasis erupted as a result of this trauma, but it has 'lived' on some areas of the scar tissue near the right temple for as long as I can remember. This area is on the meridian which connects with the Triple Warmer acupuncture point.

My partner of this time had developed a practical interest in yoga, with the resultant dietary shifts away from the norm. My emotional stability, often in one or another state of imbalance, interpreted this as a threat, as I held the new natural and 'health' foods in suspicion. Of course there was more to the new wave than yoghurt and sesame bars, wholemeal bread and muesli, and I gradually developed a general awareness of better health through eating and attitudes. With greater maturity I evolved a more open mind, but for the present I continued to cater to, and even cultivate, my tastes for rich and exotic foods, wines, restaurants, and a generally irresponsible and debauched lifestyle.

With that relationship ended I plunged into my new corporately fuelled self-esteem. Forsaking any notions of healthy eating, I replaced breakfast with three or four cups of very strong coffee gulped down with cream and sugar, and a cake or some quick combination of fat and carbohydrate grabbed on the run. Lunch was quite often begrudgingly taken at the club or hotel, in each case washed down with the inevitable couple of drinks (usually bourbon and ugly black fizz), or better still, sandwiched between time and motion studies and production schedules back at the desk. On the nights when I didn't work back, meals were usually nutritious but rich and a chef's creation, and there was always at least one bottle of wine. I favoured red wine, so at least I was getting some antioxidants!

Certainly I was burning up more nutrients through nervous energy and general bodily abuse than I was taking in, or than my body was able to manufacture in its racing duel with my destructive lifestyle. I smoked three packets of Camels a day. This was in the period 1974–75, and I was enjoying myself immensely, with a disposable income and all of the appurtenances afforded by life in an exciting city, a gorgeous, highly intelligent girlfriend, and the freedom to travel and enjoy the 'good life'. At the same time I had some excruciating piles, but probably didn't mention this to my girlfriend (she professes not to remember now).

Suddenly a planned holiday in the sun was preceded by the eruption of psoriasis all over my body. Previously there had been patches on my elbows almost constantly. My first real holiday in over a year was curtailed by the onset of an intense influenza-like feeling. In spite of the mucus rising in my head, the lure of the security of home base, and the (most important) desire to be fit and ready for return to work in a few days, led me to catch the first available jet back to Sydney (almost bursting my eardrums in the process).

That night I caught a chill which significantly worsened the already severe attack of influenza. Choosing the closest doctor's surgery next day, I consulted a fellow of about my own age, a locum as it happened, who gave me some advice which I later appreciated, although I had entered the surgery under the assumption that he would give me a remedy for a speedy recovery—i.e. an antibiotic. He refused to give me a prescription and bluntly told me, 'Go and make your own antibodies. Eat some fish, salads, food that will give you nourishment. Make yourself healthy again!'

Well, it was good advice, but I didn't act on it immediately. Instead I went into a state of withdrawal which really amounted to fasting, because I was reliant on my own ability to go out and purchase supplies—an act I wasn't really in the mood for—and anyway was confined to bed. It was another two weeks before I gained sufficient strength to make a steady return to the work that had piled up on my desk.

Soon the creativity that had made the job so enjoyable diminished. At the same time the psoriasis that had accompanied me to the Gold Coast spread all over my abdomen and chest, across my scalp, and down my back and legs. The sheer discomfort of it sent me scurrying for the first skin specialist to whom I could gain referral. I think this was the first dermatologist I had been to see since I was about twelve years old.

I was warmly greeted by a very pleasant person. She confessed that her profession was still quite puzzled by the disease and encouraged me to keep my chin up. Frankly, I hadn't expected more than this, and was less disturbed emotionally by my affliction after all these years than I was by the immense discomfort of it—like being encrusted with a taut scale, or constricted by a too-tight suit of chainmail. In fact, it was primarily to achieve relief from this and its almost incessant itching that set me enquiring after the latest 'big guns'. As the doctor supplied prescriptions and numerous repeats for an ointment and cream which were the latest and 'best available', she asked if I had been using corticosteroids, the last popular treatment. When I replied no, I hadn't, she responded, 'That's good, because American research has found that they can cause cancer of the liver.'

With my wallet considerably lighter from the encounter, I presented three prescriptions at the adjoining pharmacy. I was dismayed to discover I had acquired a small fortune's worth of acrid-smelling substances which I could bear using only a couple of times because of their odour, which I found insulting, and the hideous, alien feeling they imposed on my body. The directions for their use required smearing preparation X over all affected areas, including the scalp, before bed, washing it off in the morning shower, and replacing it with preparation Y, which was to be worn until evening. Because of the feeling they imposed, which was actually worse than the crusty body sock, and because I was in constant contact with other people in my job, for whom I felt the odour was offensive, I discontinued the regimen and suffered the normal course of the attack.

This ended as a coincidence of my getting out of the demanding job in mid-1975 and pursuing a more relaxed and less stress-oriented lifestyle, drifting into better foods and ideals. I was a fairly regular visitor to the fabulous beaches on Sydney's south and north shores. This new phase, where I also entered into self-discovery and realised a talent for writing, culminated in a move away from the city in 1977 towards healthier and happier alternatives. I still lived near the coast and made good use of the sun and surf.

Shortly after leaving the city, I quit smoking. (I took up the Camels again less than a year later, finally quitting these for good in 1987.) The event of my first attempt at quitting was celebrated by also abandoning red meats and avoiding animal-based foodstuffs. Previously I had been a great meat eater, preferring juicy rare steaks and rich sauces, so this represented quite a change—which I have never regretted making. 'Image' also became less important with this change of lifestyle. Thereafter I was without my crusty bedfellow for many months, or until emotional circumstances took a destined sidestep. I was still idealistic, even refusing to use synthesisers in the recording studio because they were incapable of harmonics, and therefore did not have a symbiotic relationship with the universal energy, the (then) 'music of the spheres'.

Inherent in my new lifestyle was the inevitability of 'paying new dues' as my former life was stripped from me, in the material sense quite literally. Under bizarre and disturbing circumstances I lost my best friend of many years, the person who was my guide and patron in a newfound profession of writing and music. For many months I lived under stressful and deprived conditions. Naturally, this invited the return of psoriasis.

These conditions were alleviated somewhat when my girlfriend of a few years before joined me. We established a home together and fairly promptly became parents. Twenty-three years later we produced this book.

While vegetarian, our diet included fresh raw cow's milk from a small dairy along the road from where we lived in a rough shack we built together.

This food was in my breakfast and coffee; I used the cream to whiten both dandelion coffee and 'real' coffee, made in a percolator. My diet was otherwise better than average, as it included fresh vegetables and no beef, lamb, pork or chicken. We lived on the coast and had plentiful supplies of fresh fish. I often baked our bread, and in general had a reputation amongst close friends for sometimes radical steadfastness in my ideals and attitudes, which were alternative to say the least. We rejected plastic packaging and as much processed food as was practicable, lived without electricity, composted, conserved and recycled—although we moved about in an old vehicle which was not particularly environmentally friendly.

* * *

When it was suggested that I rub some natural oils into the psoriasis patches that were growing larger on my legs and elbows, I found immediate relief from its itchy constriction, which gave me an enormous psychological boost. With it came a feeling of achievement from that little bit of self-help, something that I had not experienced before. With the natural oils there wasn't the smell of the steroid or tar treatments, never mind their carcinogenic contributions. (Even cod-liver oil's fishy smell was preferable to their smells.)

During a consultation my wife had with a natural healer in 1979, this man noticed psoriasis on my elbows. 'I used to have it!' he exclaimed, 'but I got rid of it very quickly with these.' He produced some tablets which he said were South African and bade me take them. His directions were to take up to four one hour before sunbathing. I never did use them, however, because I didn't know what they were or how they worked. They were probably a synthesised psoralen. Psoralen is a furocoumarin present in some vegetables and herbs. (A couple of years later, when large, burning and blistering inflammations erupted on my right shoulder, a workmate asked if I had been in contact with parsnips in the last day or so. As it happened, I had been gardening without a shirt and had harvested a couple of parsnips. The plants were very difficult to extract from the ground and I had to grip them hard at the base of the leaves. My workmate described similar experiences. I have assumed that a photosynthetic reaction occurred to produce the shingle-like symptoms. The blisters were effectively treated with the trusty pawpaw ointment, but for several months dis-pigmentation remained where the blisters had been.)

Having rejected orthodox medicine, and unable to afford treatment by many of the number of the new breed of therapists who were springing up with the New Age, I resigned myself to the inevitability of the old affliction, finding suitable but temporary relief in the natural oils. It didn't occur to me at the time to research psoriasis in the natural health literature which adorned our bookshelves, although I did learn from Adelle Davis's books about pantothenic acid deficiencies.[5] Looking back, this failure is quite remarkable—here I was, avidly pursuing a lifestyle that threw up all sorts of challenges to orthodox thought, and yet I wasn't aware of how to deal with the stuff that was on my body. I experienced how an extreme headache and the anxiety that accompanied it could be fixed with an infusion of valerian. This is the herbal (read natural) precursor of valium. I witnessed the amazing properties of comfrey in the healing of a broken toe whose owner wrapped it with a comfrey leaf poultice. At the same time, my naturally gregarious inclinations meant I had no difficulty in relating with neighbours who slaughtered and hung their own beasts.

Shortly the passage of time, the gathering of experience, and the advent of necessity brought upon by 'the way of things' drew my life towards a dramatic tangent. The full nature of the events that followed over a period of several months, and which some readers might recognise sufficiently if I describe them as a crucifixion experience or a self-initiatory, shamanistic ordeal, demand a separate and dedicated retelling. However, suffice to say that I took what was an intensely spiritual and thoroughly rewarding step, albeit life-threatening and totally disruptive to material well-being. Throughout the entire period October 1979 to February 1980 I was alone and 'in my thoughts'. Later I would come upon a wonderful little book called *The Art of Inner Listening*, and on many occasions since that time have 'consulted' my inner self on appropriate courses of action and decisions worthy of making. For those readers who do not understand what I am describing, let me just say that it was a major cleanout and a step onto a new path, and without which, if you like, I would not be writing this.

Having spent twelve weeks literally 'in the wilderness', crippled with leg ulcers and undergoing this major detoxication and rebirth, I was physically an emaciated wreck, with not a single, tangible worldly shore on which to ground. All traces of psoriasis vanished from my body during this period, although they returned with a vengeance later. I had very little contact with the world outside during my spontaneous retreat, speaking at any length with other human beings on only three occasions, all within the same week, and two of them on the same day when I was brought fresh food. In fact I hid from some visitors. Otherwise I lived off what I had in store and what was growing in the garden, a true survival experience. I remember a couple of 'meals'—one, a comfrey leaf wrapped around a ripe tomato, another a handful of rosemary and cabbage leaves chopped together with some diced capsicum.

The first person to visit me was a fellow who had led groups in internal alchemy—a process of transmutation which incorporated ritual, herbal medicines and cabbalistic practices. 'You went very deep,' he told me. He also informed me that through pursuing and succeeding at 'spontaneous initiation' I had 'reversed [my] genetic structure'. I knew that I was very much in touch with an inner voice, for it was this that had guided me in absolutely everything I did during that time and for quite a while afterwards. This is still with me, and I can call upon it whenever I want to.

So there I was in a blazing hot, dry February 1980. Enlightened, but with no money or clothes that fitted me—I weighed just over 98 pounds (45 kilograms)—I was completely out of food and most people I met, other than the few friends who thought they knew the circumstances, believed I was crazy. Because of my experience I knew quite conclusively that I was not, despite the physical appearance which suggested otherwise—festered skin-and-bone and utterly dishevelled, and still with no psoriasis. Not at any time did I consider myself to be a 'victim'. With the profound although sometimes confusing help I received from my ordeal, and which had accompanied me throughout it, I took the first tentative steps back into the world.

Suddenly the ulcers were disappearing. These were tropical leg ulcers, thought to be attributable to either the creek waters, some sort of detoxification, or inappropriate dieting. I counted 24 in all, ranging in size from a thumbnail to the palm of my hand. They had erupted from scratches and insect bites and I had not once wittingly treated them, although with hindsight I recognised several foods and herbs which my 'inner voice' directed me to eat, as being therapeutic to their healing. Nor did I experience any pain under certain conditions. Despite this lack of treatment, and the possible deep and damaging influence of the ulcerations, I have only two hardly discernible scars, each about the size of a five cent piece, as physical reminders of this otherwise indelible experience.

No sooner had the ulcers cleared away than their places were taken by psoriasis in exactly the same dimensions and configurations. However, not satisfied with adorning my legs and ankles, the tops and even arches of both feet, it appeared on my arms from the elbows down, the backs and palms of both hands in symmetry, and settled under two fingernails. The armoured breastplate returned, but this time it extended under both armpits and onto my back and buttocks, scrotum and penis, altogether lending the appearance of a now tattered and moth-eaten chainmail. The familiar fallout-prone crust again covered much of my scalp, and all in all the only parts of my body not affected were the face and ears. Yes, I felt I *was* psoriasis.

Without my recent experience and its nature, I would not have handled the new physical and emotional implications as I did. I empathise totally with the many psoriatics who have and are presently experiencing such a dreadful state of being. Confronted with a bedraggled and battered veritable skeleton in the first mirror I had consulted for months I laughed at myself, although this was more a hoarse cackle, as I recall. 'All you can do,' I told myself, 'is get out there and start again.'

With the 42 cents which represented the sum of my fortune at that time, my first contact with the world outside was an acupuncturist friend who was quite shocked and puzzled by my condition. He measured very weak pulses and almost zero energy levels, and treated these effectively with moxibustion candles and acupuncture. A severely damaged liver was diagnosed from the derangement of my big toes and a brown pigment discolouration on the inside of each thigh. His ensuing thoroughgoing treatment and intimate concern gave me immediate and long-lasting relief, plus the necessary energy for what lay ahead. His fee was the jar of fresh-picked blood plums I had taken along.

Encouraged by my recent self-reliance I had resolved to heal myself of psoriasis, believing also that it was something only I could achieve. It was paramount in importance with creating a new life for myself and, I hoped, my estranged family, who had not heard from me for three months.

Creating new family relationships took more time than I had imagined, and so I hungrily sought out all the information about psoriasis which I could find. The most I did find at the time was in Paavo Airola's book *Are You Confused?*[6] Friends also came to the rescue with specific dietary advice gained from macrobiotic and natural healing experiences. I was shown vervain, a splendid nerve tonic that grew wild, and was advised to add apple cider vinegar and tea-tree oil to the bath. The latter proved successful, but also attracted mosquitoes, even though it is used as a repellent (I have never been able to work that one out). Gradually I formulated a personal dietary program based on what I could afford, and drew up a comprehensive course of supplementary vitamins and minerals, which was less affordable. Nevertheless, things miraculously began to fall into place for me, and shortly I was well on the long road to complete recovery, although there was still some way to travel.

It must be realised that during that twelve-week 'retreat' I underwent deep and prolonged fasting—or, as a friend later put it, 'That's not fasting, that's starvation'. While overtly I appeared to be a severely depleted individual, and in a condition which was not helped by the nutritionally depleting characteristics of psoriasis, I had not undergone starvation. In the state of fasting the body is denied nutrients and obtains them from its own reserves. I had eaten very tightly controlled foods in small portions, and I had drunk fresh rainwater—there was a determined, structured and constructive process involved. Nevertheless, it was doubly essential to restore nutrients if I expected to actually achieve a healing state. I already believed that natural, preferably organic food was the best way to achieve this in the long term, and that I urgently needed lots of it. Prior to this I had held a fashionable disdain for 'taking pills'. However, faced with this new necessity I compiled the course of supplements advised by Paavo Airola, together with my own additions and adaptations gleaned from various other publications (some of which are listed in the *References* for this book). I persevered with this course of therapy for several weeks, and gradually diminished the dosages until they were no longer necessary.

To present this picture in its true perspective—as I believe it is necessary to present a life-size model for the less determined reader who is hesitant about embarking on a self-healing course—my circumstances, which already might be perceived as more radical than many readers would willingly endure, soon took another extreme course. I embarked on a 'pilgrimage' through three states and over 5,000 miles (9,000 kilometres), complete with about three weeks' supply of vitamins and many of the necessary foods. I did this for personal reasons, amongst which was a determination to spend some time working in the vineyards near Mildura in Victoria, or so I hoped (this work had been arranged on my behalf and I had committed myself). Because I was travelling by train all the way, and was therefore at the mercy of the poor food that was then made available, I deemed it efficacious to take my own along. So it was that the single piece of luggage that I carried through New South Wales to Melbourne, then to Mildura and on to Adelaide, contained about 40 pounds (18 kilograms) of prepared nourishment, herb teas, fruits, nuts, body oils and I don't know how many tablets and capsules, and not a few reference books into the bargain!

Of course, it was a nice idea to consider putting in a few days grape-picking, and I did try, eventually succeeding in picking a grand total of 147 buckets in two days. The greatest benefit came in the form of the luscious fruits with their fresh juice and vitamins, the exercise in the sun, the camaraderie of the itinerant pickers, and the chance to earn a few dollars to maintain supplement stocks. However, I was only hurting myself further by persevering, and on a very hot morning I walked out to the highway and hitchhiked to Adelaide.

Since embarking on my self-healing I had been oiling myself at least twice daily. The directions were again from Paavo Airola. The blend I prepared for myself was a 50:50 combination of apricot kernel and sesame oils. I know what it is like to oil large areas of psoriasis. It takes time; you have to consider factors such as clothing, furniture, going to work. The oil becomes cloudy and little bits of dead skin proliferate through it.

It is possible that my strenuous and idealistic efforts were only prolonging the attack, as I was still an emotional mess and found it difficult to maintain the rigid diet. Aided by a couple of days work in Adelaide, I caught a bus direct to Sydney where, I had decided, I would consult the Dorothy Hall Institute for whose founder I had a profound respect and admiration. Late that February I arrived in Sydney and was very fortunate to be granted a short consultation with one of her colleagues that same afternoon, shortly before I was due to catch the train north. The short consultation became quite a lengthy one. As I was still only a few weeks into my self-appointed healing regimen, imagine my delight and encouragement at learning through iridiagnosis that although I was still slightly deficient in vitamin C, had a circulatory problem, and was still having difficulty producing sufficient enzymes, I was otherwise nutritionally sound! As problems with enzymes and circulation are symptomatic of psoriasis, it could be deduced that my self-healing was otherwise on target, provided I increased the intake of vitamin C.

Rosehip tea was prescribed for this, and celery seed tea and alfalfa sprouts for circulation and enzymes respectively. My spleen was also damaged. I was told how disruption to this organ, which plays a vital role in developing immunities and in the formation of the blood and the breakdown of old blood cells, would explain my feeling at the time of being 'all over the place', because the spleen also represents our 'earth', or how firmly our feet 'are placed on the ground'. Certainly mine were not at the time; I was yearning for stability and direction. Comfrey was prescribed to correct this, and for the psoriasis I was given a homeopathic or herbal preparation which I faithfully administered orally for the prescribed course of about twelve weeks.

Incidentally, the iridiagnosis also confirmed that a residue of toxins still had to be eliminated. Whether this was achieved through the bout of psoriasis which still had some weeks to run is uncertain. What is certain is that in the years since I have undoubtedly been pouring in more toxins, through diet which has lapsed from time to time, or through not regularly detoxicating.

The Dorothy Hall clinic practises wholistic medicine, wherein specific attention is devoted to the whole person and the treatment is determined for the individual rather than through a blanket cure, which orthomolecular practitioners know to be an erroneous application of the healing gifts. The body will heal itself with the right help—nothing will 'cure' it. The preparation which was made up for me was specially formulated for me and my condition, and thus might have less effect on another individual. I have found this individuality to be one of the most important aspects of treatment and believe only in therapists who reflect it in practice.

My consultant spent a lot of time listening to descriptions of the detoxifying retreat. She enquired whether I had considered hypnotherapy as a healing form. I replied that I had recently read of its benefits in treating emotional and psychosomatic illnesses, categories in which many practitioners place psoriasis. This strikes me as a cop-out on their part. I think they are overcome by the nature of disease and incapable of coming to terms with its diverse physiological implications, either through tunnel-vision training or an inability to perceive their profession as other than egalitarian. Nevertheless that is their problem, providing they do not impose their misconceptions on sufferers who consult them in good faith, for it is little better than declaring that the patient suffers from an incurable disease. At best it might indicate that the patient is the better doctor. By no means do I wish to rubbish the orthodox professions, however, because my greatest help was yet to come from this quarter.

The consultant concluded the session with a referral to a GP who practised hypnotherapy. I telephoned the doctor and gave him a brief description of the circumstances. He suggested I spend a 'week of lunchtimes' with him at a future date; I made a note of this and headed north.

In March 1980 I became involved with many other people in an effort to save an area of beach and headland from being sand-mined. I joined an on-site camp by the sea, thereby taking advantage of the sun and seawater. Members of two indigenous Australian tribes, the Gumbangerii and Dunghatti, whose tribal origins lay on the very beach we were attempting to save, joined the camp. They were very adept at catching fish and preparing them in delightful ways; generally the lifestyle in this hastily convened community was most conducive to my emotional and constitutional up-building. I lament the loss of the innocence of those days.

On the very first day of the camp, as some of us sat around the fire, me with my lesions plain to all eyes, an Aboriginal woman surprised me with the declaration that her grandfather had had psoriasis. 'He used to boil the bark of that tree,' she said, pointing to a nearby tree that she named the bloodwood. Apparently he applied the infusion directly to the lesions. I had never before considered that indigenous people would suffer from the disease, but of course this is not to say that they would have prior to the Europeans' arrival. I did not try making the infusion, however.

I was experiencing difficulty with soap, in those straitened times probably a relatively cheap oatmeal-based variety. Whether or not the scale was removed, no amount of rinsing would remove the waxy soap film from the psoriatic lesions. I quickly concluded that no soap was best, and later modified this by using liquid castile, but only on unaffected areas. It was necessary to use the castile on my scalp (as a shampoo), but I can offer no conclusion about its effects, adverse or otherwise. I was not oiling my scalp at this time.

On April 9 I rejoined my family in their new home further up the coast, therefore gaining an enormous psychological boost. My skin had significantly improved but I still felt some way from total healing. Fortunately my weight had increased, and all but a few patches of psoriasis on my upper torso had cleared, although many still remained on my legs. Deborah insisted on oiling my scalp for me each night.

At this time our circle of friends included a young woman from California who confessed to not being able to cook. Her mother had never taught her, and it transpired that this was regarded as a perfectly natural sequence of events. The family had eaten prepared foods; fresh produce and the home-cooked meal were quite out of the ordinary. This was in 1980. I remember also when another friend stayed with a family on Long Island in 1975. She spoke of meals which consisted of one or another frozen or similarly pre-prepared concoction nuked in the microwave. The somewhat cavernous refrigeration system contained absolutely zero fresh food items. This is normal practice and obviously has been for decades. What chance then for a society to suddenly turn on a generation or two of practice and decide to eat food? What chance the rest of the world too, with populaces of all ages and persuasions, succumbing to the proliferation of dietary habits in the form of more fast-food (fast-fat) chains?

Meanwhile I remembered the hypnotherapist in Sydney. In April I was in the doctor's rooms and benefiting from my first experience with hypnotherapy. He began by asking whether I knew anything about Transactional Analysis, a method of identifying and dealing with unstable emotional conditioning, published in the bestselling paperback *I'm OK,*

You're OK by Thomas A. Harris MD. I knew a little about it but had not read the book, so the doctor lent me a copy. Over the next few days I learned much about myself and applied the information contained in this book. For the first time I was given a very effective insight into long overdue psychological healing.

Then came my first practical experience in hypnotherapy. As I lay on the couch and the doctor bade me relax and allow the peripheral thoughts to chase one another around my descending consciousness, a feeling of relaxation came over me, similar to that afforded by some of the massages I had enjoyed at the anti-sand mining camp. The first session was short, needfully so as it was an introduction for both of us: for me, because my only other experience with hypnotism had been the theatrical tricks that are not hypnotherapy, and which have little place in healing other than to incite laughter; for the doctor, because he had to learn about his patient and my particular needs. Already, however, I was feeling more positive, and as I left the surgery after only 45 minutes I genuinely felt that I was getting somewhere.

The doctor asked me what I wanted to achieve from the proposed sessions. He also asked me to think about my family and my life, and to let whatever emotions this triggered to flow freely to the surface. In this respect he was also approaching treatment from a wholistic viewpoint, and clearly worked with the individual patient to identify a desired outcome and jointly establish a goal.

I saw the doctor during his lunchbreak each day for five days. As our sessions progressed I was gradually taken deeper and with each session another level was revealed to me. Those who are unfamiliar with hypnotherapy will be interested to learn that the subject remains wholly conscious, and that it is the deeper subconscious that is brought to the surface. The deeper one goes, the deeper the levels of subconscious that are tapped. It is like a recording tape buried in a time capsule: the information stored on the tape can be modified or wiped; the subconscious can reveal all because it forgets nothing. In my case, I wanted to know the root cause of my condition, why I had it and what lay in my past to make this affliction necessary. Perhaps this was too esoteric for the practical scientist, for we never explored this avenue.

It does raise an interesting question, though. While the human mind is born with a certain amount of inherited knowledge (the desire for breast milk and knowing where to find it, the knowledge of appropriate responses to pain and pleasure), as adults we possess more knowledge that is learned through experience (or memory) than is based on innate neuronal connections. Knowledge stored in the brain increases for the first 39 years of life, after which it gradually decreases (cf. the limbic system's role in emotions, as discussed in *Part 1*).

Although the root cause of the psoriasis had not revealed itself, I was given a tool with which I could rapidly remove all traces of the disease from my body in a very short time. Even during that week in Sydney I could already see results.

The method was simply this: 'You have,' I was told under hypnosis, 'the power to instruct your body to heal itself. Your body doesn't want this stuff all over it, tell it to get rid of it. Your body will. It is only waiting for you to take control. You know what you want, tell your body to carry it out for you and it will.'

What could be simpler? I was to practise this technique as often as I wished or felt the need. It simply required me to lie comfortably and relax completely. As I slipped deeper into relaxation and my subconscious rose to the surface—while all the time I remained conscious and alert—I was to visualise the psoriasis vanishing from my body to be replaced with healthy, clear skin. This technique also replenished my scattered self-esteem. The net result was to correct my posture, giving me a profound air of certainty and confidence, and an indelible glow of happiness and security. The 'new me' was plainly visible to the friends with whom I stayed for the time, and the patches were already diminishing in size and severity.

On the fifth day the doctor surprised me by saying that I was ready to return to my family and, further, that today's session would improve my technique so that I could use it to help others. And so, armed with this magnificent relaxation and healing tool, I returned to the North Coast where I delighted in continuing with the practice of self-hypnosis, topical oiling and dietetic therapies.

By this time my supplementary intake was down to a trickle as my diet was now adequate. The rapid improvement afforded by the hypnotherapy also meant that only a couple of weeks remained before my skin was completely clear. By June no traces remained anywhere on my body.

In early August, while in Sydney with my family, we visited the doctor to extend our gratitude. I showed him my tanned and healthy legs. 'It's a miracle!' he exclaimed, denying any part he had played in, or reason to claim for my success. Without Dr Kos Aroney's help, I would not have cleared up so rapidly. He was a true healer and humanitarian, and I owe much to him.

Self-hypnosis

By 1982, I had come to the conclusion that the greatest contribution to the two years of dramatic remission I had enjoyed was hypnotherapy, wherein I learned that I had control over my body and how to use it. I had undergone an extreme detoxification before the psoriasis erupted; the dietary and supplementary regimens were even more necessary in view of the severe debility—and heaven knows, all readers would benefit from improved dietetics—however, the most rapid and visible achievements were gained once I undertook hypnotherapy. I have to admit, however, that for the next fourteen years I hardly ever practised self-hypnosis and on many occasions and for prolonged periods of time ignored my own dietary advice.

A decade or so after my encounter with Dr Aroney, my son had misplaced an important item. I offered to hypnotise him because, as I explained, his subconscious would remember where he had placed it. He agreed, and in the hypnotic state I gave the instruction that, upon being brought out of the hypnotic state, he would go immediately to where he had left the item. He did just that.

The mind is indeed a wonderful and mysterious entity—I believe our most important possession in this (third dimensional) state. It can be a tricky companion, though. Someone once asked me, 'Do you ever suffer from writer's block?' 'There is no such thing,' I replied. 'It is automatically overcome by starting to write—anything. I write anything, the first thing that comes to mind and that is the process of beginning. This might never be used in subsequent drafts, but it is the best way of ignoring the mind's efforts to trick you into thinking you are stumped for an idea.'

I don't believe that it is necessary to fully understand the mind in order to have it work for us; more a case of adopting a positive outlook. In this respect the conscious, subconscious and mind are separate though connected entities. I have a fairly definite view of what the mind is—which probably wouldn't sit very well with orthodoxy, but that's neither here nor there. Ultimately, I believe too much understanding can cloud the ability to get on with it.

One of my favourite books, *The Mind Parasites* by Colin Wilson, has a gathering of earth's scientists seizing control of the moon with their unified thought power and flinging it out of our solar system. (Because it houses some shitty entities who have been sapping the intellect of Earth's inhabitants since the Dark Ages. Sound familiar?) This book is a favourite for several reasons—I love the concept, it is a remarkably original piece of work, and in

1976, without having ever read it (my first experience of it being in 1979), I wrote a radio play with a storyline and characters which are eerily similar. Is the individual mind merely a spoon-dip into a soup bowl after all?

I believe our thought power could be the greatest power we possess. To create a thought is to create energy. Furthermore, to visualise something is to create that event or act in other parts of reality (why stop at one?).

Familiar themes

In my experience, suffering with psoriasis to the extent I did was in very large measure the result of a lack of sensible, lucid information and education about the simplicity of dis-ease—in particular psoriasis—and in its place much unjustified mystery and misery; thus denying easy relief to many.

The roles of diet and proper elimination, positive and stress-free lifestyles, and a happy life-outlook, are unquestionable in my interpretation of balanced health. In those days, however, despite pursuing an ideology that offered many avenues of recourse to adequate health and balance, I was still seriously afflicted. This must underscore the fine line that exists between adequate and *essential* individual nutrition.

A positive approach required belief in myself, dismissal of the concept of blame, and assertion of my right to individuality. I had long regarded blanket rules designed for a mass as unwholesome and in many instances immoral, such as enforced vaccination of infants and children and the fluoridation of water supplies. Where these ideologies go wrong is in asserting that 'this' is right for absolutely everyone. This process denies individual free will. To declare that everyone will now be forced to eat organic vegetarian food would be equally wrong; it denies choice, personal power and individuality. It is plainly stupid for a civilisation that purports to be advancing to eradicate the individual in favour of the herd mentality, but that is clearly what is at hand.

My subconscious retains the key to my hereditary or conditioned weaknesses. Being personally satisfied with the proof of dietary, metabolic and toxic factors in psoriasis affliction, I am interested in further research into the central nervous system, and neurobiological and subconscious factors. Indeed, might I predict that greater research breakthroughs will be achieved once researchers and practitioners accept the necessity for wholistic and orthomolecular approaches, which will enable more time and effort to be devoted to neurobiological-oriented considerations. I believe this to be far more relevant and important than genetic research, and wholeheartedly more ethical.

January 2001

Today I feel great. A very real and positive outcome of my research for this book has been the rekindling of the desire to tidy up my dietary habits. I have been practising what I am reading and writing about (as you would!). My typical daily diet now begins with fresh fruits in the morning and some dandelion coffee. I have just had a bowl of delicious muesli, something I ordinarily wouldn't consider because of the need to accompany it with cow's milk or soy milk. Instead I used oat milk. This is made by soaking and blending organic rolled oats in water. The milky liquid so produced is sweet and has, well, an oaty flavour. Organic rolled oats, chopped almonds, freshly pounded sunflower seeds, linseed, rice bran, some chopped Chinese dates and organic apple make a fabulous muesli. Some mind-blowing coffee and carbohydrate lift the morning, and lunch is often a large salad with a seed oil, sprinkled with roasted sunflower seeds and the roasted sesame seed and sea salt mixture described in *Part III: Taking Control*. The sweet tooth that inevitably emerges in mid-afternoon is satisfied with whatever comes to hand. There might be another coffee or some black tea in the afternoon too, although this is much less likely in summer. An iced dandelion coffee is good at these times. Dinner is cooked vegetables, sometimes organic chicken breast (but only the breast; the part which provides most protein) with fresh herbs from the garden, rice, pesto or a chick pea dish. Dessert simply doesn't figure in our household and hasn't for many years, nor has coffee or tea after the meal. A white or red wine might accompany dinner and it's rare that the bottle isn't finished afterwards. I usually cook at least one fish or seafood dish on the weekend.

The dietary/digestive implications of leaky gut syndrome are of particular interest to me today. In a future book, I intend to elaborate on some specific tests which I will undertake to explore this syndrome.

While I am using several different topical applications, and alternating them in no particular pattern, the best thing I have been doing for several months is to take clay and spirulina regularly. The clay in particular, I believe, is responsible for a generally calming effect on the (albeit small) elbow patches, in addition to the renewal of lost minerals. (Both clay and *Cyanobacteria* are presented in detail in *Part III: Taking Control*.) A small jar of vitamin A oil is very effective; 1000IU of Retinol palmitate with vitamin E antioxidant in a safflower oil base costs about A\$23 for 1 oz (50 ml); it is a pleasure to use, and quite economical, very light so a little goes a long way. Retinol (vitamin A) cream is only available with a doctor's prescription. I have also experimented with vitamin E cream and hemp oil.

All of these are beneficial to the restoration of elasticity and suppleness in the few small spots (elbows, one shin). The vitamin E cream (concentrated, high-potency) has been particularly good: it produces a very lasting result. I noticed on several occasions that if I apply it to my elbows last thing at night, there are no scales formed by next morning. The hemp product is also excellent. Nowhere else have I intentionally stated a brand name and neither would I endorse a product without careful consideration. I do recommend the vendor of the hemp product, The Body Shop. This international organisation, which is British in origin, practises with a conscionable business philosophy and commitment to the community, and sells some good products. Hemp Body Butter is amongst them. It contains hemp seed oil, lanolin and babassu oil (produced from the nut of a tree native to Brazil). Another, Hemp Well Oiled, is a combination of sweet almond oil, hemp seed oil and sesame oil, a versatile lotion suitable for surface treatment and adding to the bath. A further reason for mentioning The Body Shop is its Community Trade policy of purchasing natural ingredients (as used in these two products) and accessories from poor or disadvantaged communities, in reciprocal relationships based on trust and respect. I have been alternating the hemp butter with a home preparation containing aloe, coconut butter and wheat germ oil that leaves the treated area feeling very cool and soothed.

The small patches on my elbows remain in what I regard as a 'benign' state, that is, uninflamed, with little or no redness, and no scale having formed in the ensuing hours; and this during some times of imbibing alcohol at a succession of parties and drinking coffee daily. The intervening holiday period (Christmas and New Year) in particularly hot and humid weather has meant lots of alcohol, especially beer (not a good drop for the likes of me) and foods I would not normally eat. Working on this book has been an absolute joy, with the attendant creative experience (and the stresses and strains of not a few long days and late nights!). A morning's escape to the beach with terrific sun exposure and swims in the ocean had the elbow patches on the run by next day. Now that this book is wrapped, a full week in the sun and surf will set the tone for the year ahead.

My scalp is virtually clear, the only treatment at the moment being some coconut oil or lavender oil massaged in occasionally (Deborah likes this too, as it helps her sleeping pattern). Some years ago, a hairdresser referred me to a brand of treatment shampoo which contains jojoba and other natural ingredients, but which also contains a bunch of chemicals. This was effective for a time, although it hardly meets the essential criteria. I have also used a plantolin-based brand which contains purified water, coco-betaine derived from coconut oil, glycerine, citric acid, plantolin extract, lavender oil, geranium oil, tea-tree oil, ylang ylang oil, but also methyl hydroxybenzoate and sodium laureth sulfate. For several weeks I have used an excellent home-made shampoo of aloe vera extract and a pure shampoo base. A sprig of rosemary from the garden is suspended in this. Interestingly, the aloe vera was purchased in 1982 when I was marketing *So-ri-a-sis*. I feel that this is the best shampoo I have ever used.

There is a basket of supplements at the breakfast bench and I sometimes use C, B complex, E, evening primrose oil, selenium and others (e.g. zinc, gingko biloba) in no particular pattern. As a result of this research, I have a large glass of spirulina at about 11 am. This—affectionately known as algae (*Aljee!*)—in combination with the fruit breakfast, has made an amazing difference to energy levels and alertness, particularly in the afternoon when the biorhythms are at their lowest ebb, and in the evening. I intend to continue with Aljee indefinitely. As with anything I have tried over the years, the initial and sometimes ongoing revulsion/hesitation/acquired taste is more than worth it for the very real benefits.

So I'm breaking rules, just as nine out of ten of us are bound to do. Perfection is not something I am seeking or necessarily capable of achieving. Nevertheless, I am able to enjoy a quality of life with and without psoriasis.

Freedom

In an 'information age' there can be no excuse for uninformedness.

In our circumstances, freedom from dis-ease is no further away than useful and worthwhile knowledge and the will to explore it.

PART III

Taking control

If we want to return to health
we must expect to change.

Bach Flower Remedies

5 Which treatment?

What's in a name?

When mainstream medicine is referred to in this book, the term 'orthodox' is applied.

In recent times 'traditional' has been used when referring to mainstream—read orthodox—medical practice. Traditional medicine is that which has been and is practised by indigenous races and by practitioners of orthomolecular, complementary or wholistic medicine—read alternative—who apply principles such as those of naturopathy (established by Hippocrates c. 400 BC), herbalism (which in many instances has as long a history as indigenous or traditional medicine or healing practice), Chinese and Ayurvedic medicine, and wholistic therapy (which as the term suggests is not a holiness but the co-operative endeavours of patient and practitioner, and takes into account mind, body and environment). It is considered presumptuous to apply the term 'traditional' to a system that cannot claim a long and successful history.[1]

Which treatment?

Whether one employs orthodox or alternative help, the prognosis varies with the individual, as work, habitat, climate, family and past history, and general state of mind all play a part. Paramount among these is the general health or constitution of the individual.

First attacks of psoriasis, particularly in children, should be nipped in the bud by employing the least stressful and non-intoxicating therapies. Because of the presence of constitutional and nervous system factors, topical and anti-symptomatic treatments on their own are inadequate and afford only temporary remissions. Insightful therapy will also look first for toxaemia, acidosis, nervous instability, gastrointestinal disorders including metabolic insufficiencies, and endocrine derangement.

Topical applications, when they are naturally derived, are invaluable for restoring flexibility and elasticity to cracked and painful skin. Overall, however, the problem with all topical applications is their limited penetrative qualities—the upper skin layer (epidermis) is partially absorbent but the dermis is not. Creams or lotions intended to heal degeneration in the lower skin layers cannot penetrate deeply enough without the assistance of a transport. Vitamin A is used in some emollients to enable delivery. This is a very important point in the use of surface applications which are intended to provide some healing properties to the lower dermis, as opposed to those which are intended merely to repair flexibility and ease the removal of a flaky crust.

Curiously, some proprietary topical applications use anti-freeze as an accelerant to enable the absorption of drugs into the epidermis.[2]

Common orthodox treatments

Orthodox therapy favours topical and ingested drug treatments that are synthetically based, and stipulates close and consistent monitoring. The modality's motivation is undoubtedly to address patients' urgent demand for easy relief from visible embarrassment and worry, and relief from pain and discomfort.

Central to this approach is gaining a reduction in keratinocyte differentiation using keratoplastic agents or keratolytic remedies. Drugs and surface applications are intended to promote healthier cornification of the epidermis, and to return to normal the chemical changes that the cells are undergoing. On the surface, chrysarobin, ichthyol, pyrogallol, resorcin, salicylic acid, sulphur and coal tar have all had their day in this spotlight.

Topical treatments

Dithranol and coal tar are still widely prescribed because they have been found to be the most effective dermatological treatments. These are prescribed for the treatment of stable plaque; tar, with PUVA and etretinate (a vitamin A compound) is used against extensive or widespread stable plaque. Weak tar preparations are used as an alternative to emollients applied to erupting guttate psoriasis.

Dithranol (synthesised chrysarobin) replaced the raw drug (chrysarobin, a plant extract) because the original was found to be a strong irritant. A substitute had to be found because chrysarobin discoloured hair and skin, caused conjunctivitis, and rotted clothing and hospital linen. Its application burnt off the psoriasis, leaving the skin white. Dithranol was found to be less of an irritant, stained skin less deeply, and did not rot fabric—although it does stain. It is likely to burn or otherwise irritate sensitive skin. Dithranol has been used as an alternative to PUVA and etretinate for treating extensive stable plaque sites. Some people experience adverse reactions to dithranol, when it is replaced by aqueous crystal violet.

Crude coal tar has anti-itch properties, makes the body sensitive to light, and contains cresol, phenol and toluene. In mixtures with zinc paste, either in its natural state or diluted with acetone or benzene, tar has been used for decades in soap and unguent forms. Coal tar is also combined with salicylic acid in a widely known and often effective ointment. Its odour and messy characteristics can be deterrents and exacerbate a delicate psychological position. Salicylic acid, once derived from willow bark and now synthesised from phenol, is an anti-inflammatory. (Coal tar is also used as a food colouring agent.)

Other varieties of tar—or oils—used in psoriasis treatments are derived from birch, beech and pine trees, and juniper berries. Coal tar usually has an alkaline reaction, wood tars an acid reaction. Larch pine is a natural source of oils or tars which are commonly and widely used against skin disorders, including psoriasis and eczema.

Orthodox medicine also offers vitamin D patches, vitamin A creams, vitamin A acid (retinoic acid), and retinoids (such as etretinate).

Dr H. C. A. Vogel, citing experience in his Swiss clinic, notes the intractability of the disease in patients who had formerly endured extensive tar and sulphur treatment, and also the very poor chances of achieving healing when patients had been given radiation treatment, which he warns against ever resorting to.[3]

Irradiation by artificial ultraviolet light A (UVA) is applied in combination with a synthesised psoralen (P), a furocoumarin, to produce a photochemical reaction which is aimed at inhibiting the cell division. Psoralens occur naturally in the body to make the skin sensitive to light. They have a very long history of human usage—the Egyptians ingested a psoralen to make the body more sensitive to ultraviolet A rays. It is thought the ultraviolet treatments disable the immune system's lymphocytes that are driving the psoriasis. Inadequate preparation or monitoring, over-treatment and photo-sensitisation can result in side-effects such as cataracts, redness (erythema), itching, blistering and darkened pigmentation. Long-term side-effects include premature ageing of the skin, carcinomas and malignant melanomas.

Many people find great convenience in ultraviolet light B (UVB) therapy. The application of what is essentially artificial sunlight is very popular in Europe and Scandinavia. This therapy is not necessarily for everyone, but those who derive genuine relief of psoriasis following exposure to natural sunlight tend to benefit the most.

Systemic treatments

Cytotoxic drugs are prescribed for oral application in severe cases, such as acute erythrodermic, unstable or generalised pustular psoriasis. These synthesised agents reduce the dramatically accelerated cellular reproduction. While these drugs are very effective, amongst their potential side-effects are chronic damage to the blood-forming organs, and to the kidneys and liver. As the proper functioning of these organs is vital to clear, healthy skin, individuals contemplating cytotoxin treatment should first determine their system's ability to cope. Furthermore, these drugs suppress or reduce the division and production of cells indiscriminately, thus they suppress the healing cells produced by the body along with the targeted cells. People who take cytotoxic drugs must abstain from alcohol and avoid conception for six months after taking them. Methotrexate is one such systemic immunosuppressive drug which is often prescribed. It is an enemy of folic acid and a powerful impediment to the enzymes necessary for DNA synthesis.

Corticosteroids are administered in tablet forms, in ointments and creams. Corticosteroids are naturally occurring chemicals or hormones secreted by the adrenal gland. The synthesised variety in tablets are clean and easy to use, whereas topical preparations can be messy, pungent, and of little psychological benefit. Acitretin or a potent steroid paste are used to treat pustular psoriasis of the hands and feet. A hydrocortisone ointment is prescribed for facial psoriasis. Steroids and antifungal agents are used against flexural psoriasis. Steroids, whether administered orally or topically, are only suppressive and will not clear the affliction at its roots nor heal any imbalance within.

Immune-suppressive drugs have also been used. Cyclosporin, used to prevent rejection after organ transplants, used in a high enough dose has been known to completely clear psoriasis. It also produces significant side-effects: it ruins the kidneys and causes high cholesterol levels.

Close monitoring of the use of such treatments is essential because people using steroids can become dependent on them, will require progressively higher doses to maintain their suppressive action, and are exposed to the well-documented side-effects.

Corticosteroid medicines and injections are even more likely to be accompanied by side-effects. Amongst these are stomach ulcers, wasting of the muscles, water retention and rapid and unwieldy weight gain, bone disintegration, further skin disorders, susceptibility to viral, bacterial and fungal infections; plus loss of periods, headaches, diabetes, growth retardation, and manic depressive and other neurological, mental and psychological disturbances.

Synthetic neurological or biological drugs are often developed from analogues of chemicals that occur naturally within the human body.

Treating emotional factors
Referral to psychological and even psychiatric help is available. Some practitioners also advocate relaxation, meditation and similar lifestyle-oriented therapies, while others offer hypnotherapy.

Prognosis
The general prognosis is that psoriatic patients suffer from a chronic and incurable disease for which there are a variety of synthesised and naturally-based remissive agents. Suggestions are offered on how to live comfortably with the disease.

6 On the surface— reversing losses, promoting healthy growth

Out, damned spot! Out, I say!

William Shakespeare, Macbeth

Our psoriatic skin is regenerating far too quickly, causing extraordinary losses of vitamins and minerals. The dry, unyielding patches can be turned into moisturised, flexible skin which is ready for the absorption of nutrients.

We must approach ourselves with great sensitivity and caring. Certainly healing elements must be applied to the skin, but they should not be in any way artificial. We must be able to participate in our healing with confidence.

Surface healing

Surface healing is important, but it must be accompanied by considerations of individual constitution and history. The treatment of skin diseases, particularly psoriasis, should always be undertaken on other levels in conjunction with surface treatment.

The most immediate requirement is a positive mental outlook, the decision by the healer to win. Nevertheless, the most immediate and obvious relief, and a resulting psychological boost, is gained by treating the ailing skin surface. This can be achieved through a very pleasant regime which quickly becomes a routine one can look forward to, for the alternatives to unpleasant synthetic agents which impose a second-rate feeling are a sunny variety of gentle, effective and subtly fragrant helpers.

The purpose of applying oils or creams is fourfold:

- **Cleansing** We want to remove the decayed cells and eliminated toxins, and to make it easier and less painful to peel away the plaque.
- **Soothing** We want to reduce discomfort, lubricate dry skin and restore elasticity, and eliminate itching and soreness.
- **Healing** We want to introduce back into the skin some of the vanishing nutrients and elements to counteract the degeneration.
- **Self-caring** We want to stimulate the practice of self-caring. Our self-esteem is greater if we don't smell like a sulphur furnace or coal pit, proclaiming disease. It is more beneficial to exude a subtle or exotic fragrance, or none at all. More importantly, we are participating in our healing and by spending time massaging natural oils into our bodies, and having friends do the areas we can't reach, we are learning about our body/ailment, and thereby obtaining more benefits than we might realise.

Natural oils and creams

Vegetable and seed oils, nut oils, and herb-based creams satisfy the criteria for surface treatment. Natural oils will provide the vitamins A, D, E and F (essential fatty acids). Oils or creams which contain vitamin E—especially wheat germ oil—activate the microcirculation at the skin surface. Any one, or a blend, of the following oils will be beneficial: sunflower seed, safflower seed, wheat germ, fletan, cod liver, linseed (flaxseed), avocado, sesame, apricot kernel and almond.

Other oils and lotions whose properties have been found to be beneficial include: vitamin A oil or cream, vitamin E oil or cream, cajuput, gotu kola, jojoba, lavender and products from the Dead Sea.

(See also *Table 2* in *Appendix 2*.)

METHOD OF APPLICATION Apply your choice of oil(s) gently and liberally to the affected parts night and morning, or as often as appears necessary. Be aware of clothing contact with the oiled areas to avoid ruining garments with staining or discolouring.

If the plaque is particularly thick and crusty, the oil as applied might not be sufficient to remove all of the crust. It might also be necessary, and indeed beneficial, to use some method of removing this either as a part of the oil's application or preceding it. Not so long ago, we were instructed to remove the plaque with a vigorous scrub with a nail brush.[1] Today we can avail ourselves of some gentler alternatives. The Scandinavian loofah is one. This can be purchased in glove form. The loofah's natural fibre has a wonderfully exfoliating effect and represents another gentle method of getting in touch with our skin surface and therefore promoting a positive mental attitude about our body and our self.

BE SELECTIVE, AND CHECK INGREDIENTS We should buy only those oils packaged in steel or brown glass labelled cold-pressed. Any oil other than that which is obtained through cold pressing is unsuitable. Non cold-pressed oils are usually extracted and processed at very high temperatures that destroy the very nutrients we are intending to derive from them, while clear glass admits light which oxidises the contents. Oils packaged in plastic are not ideal, nor are so-called 'vegetable' oils or 'blended vegetable' oils, as these can contain cotton seed oil (with high concentrations of pesticides and similar toxins) or oils from genetically modified (GM) or similarly unnatural sources. Many commercial brands of 'vegetable' oils have some mineral oil content, which will remove fat-soluble vitamins from the skin. Mineral oil destroys vitamin D; D and A are the only vitamins which are easily absorbed into the deeper layers of the skin. 'Baby oil' is mineral based. Likewise avoid any oil or preparation which is perfumed, unless you know the scent to be benign, that is, derived directly from a herb or plant, such as lavender (also see *Soaps* and *Shampoos*, pages 131–132). Olive oil is fine providing it is fresh virgin olive oil, cold-pressed and packaged in steel or brown glass.

Check product labels thoroughly. When you see '100% pure', the element you want might well be 100 per cent pure in the product, but it might be merely one ingredient in a formula that includes many other substances, generally preservatives and stabilisers. Read the fine print. This is especially important to ensure that a 'natural' product does not introduce an irritation or allergic reaction. The same is true of any product which is intended for surface application or ingestion.[2]

Other natural skin treatments
ALLANTOIN   This is simply a cell-multiplier, which works in a similar principle to the process of keratinocytosis in so far as the replacement of body cells is accelerated; the difference being that allantoin speeds up the natural

rate of cell proliferation and alleviates irritation. Native Americans used it to cicatrise their wounds. The root of the herb comfrey is a natural source of allantoin. It is available in a number of ointment and cream preparations and can be used in its raw state. Similarly, bruises, boils, and ulcerous wounds will respond favourably to a comfrey poultice, because of the many other medicinal properties of the plant (see next section under *Herbs*, pages 145–149 for further details of comfrey's nutritive values, and also *Poultices, Packs and Pelotherapy*, below). Synthetically prepared allantoin powder has been used in preparations to stimulate the formation of surface epithelial skin cells.

ALOE VERA Renowned for its healing properties and benefits to ailing skin, aloe vera can be obtained in gel and liquid form. Preference should be given to 100 per cent plant extract. As with any new topical application tried for the first time, first apply a small amount to evaluate your skin's reaction to it. While some psoriatics report success with aloe vera, others find it an irritant. It is the aloin, the active principle in the juice, which provides aloe's anti-inflammatory and wound healing benefits. The pulp or gel is 96 per cent water. The other 4 per cent contains the polysaccharides glucose and mannose, and other trace elements. This combination of water and carbohydrates can be beneficial to the penetrative action that is necessary for the transport of healing components in topical emollients, creams, lotions and gels.

AVOCADO OIL Added to the bath, this can leave the skin with a luxuriant lustre.

BERGAMOT OIL Applied prior to oiling with other substances, bergamot oil has been found by many people to be beneficial. However, please see the notes on *Photosensitivity*, page 134.

CALENDULA OFFICINALIS Available as calendula cream and calendula oil (infused variety), this is highly effective as a surface treatment. It combines well with comfrey and hypericum as a soothing healer and promotes wound reparation without scarring. See *Herbs*, pages 145–149, for more herbs for internal and external application.

CHLOROPHYLL Derived from both alfalfa and fresh-water algal sources, chlorophyll is added to cosmetics and food, on the one hand for its therapeutic applications and on the other as a colouring agent. Its use is legendary in diverse circles including the battlefields of war—it was applied to disinfect wounds and prevent infection during World War I. (See also *Chlorophyll*, page 142.)

GERMAN CHAMOMILE This is used in the manufacture of an ointment which is effective in helping to repair skin damage caused by psoriasis. Soothing topical treatments of chamomile can be easily prepared as a wash or compress. Chamomile's therapeutic properties can be largely attributed to the cutaneous absorption of its major active principle, levomenol, or sesquiterpenic alcohol, and the anti-inflammatory action of the oliogenous substances azulene and chamazulene.

HEMP OIL In its (officially legal) industrial strength variety, hemp oil is right at the top of natural sources of the essential fatty acid omega-6.

LIQUORICE ROOT Powdered or in extract form used in a cream or lotion, this softens the skin and reduces inflammation.

PAPAYA (PAWPAW) OINTMENT Relieves, cleanses and promotes healing for cuts, abrasions, eczema and dermatitis.

POULTICES, PACKS AND PELOTHERAPY The beneficial application of herbs, clay, mud or kelp directly to the skin's surface has been around for as long as the skin has suffered wounds. Oils and herbs can be used for drawing inflammation and irritation, indeed toxins from the body and its organs. The use of facial and body mud packs in beauty therapy is intended to draw impurities from the skin, to improve circulation, and to impart beneficial nutrients. For the psoriatic, the aim is to draw impurities from the affected site in addition to restoring lost minerals. Patience is required, but the results will make it all worthwhile.

Generally, a poultice using an oil is made by first warming the oil to blood temperature, and smearing it thoroughly over the area to be treated. This is covered with brown paper or a cloth (of a natural fabric only), and plastic wrap used to seal the wrapping tight. It is then best to rest with this fastened for an hour or so—in the sun is ideal, as it is necessary to keep warm.

Any of the oils listed above, as well as castor oil, can be used either alone or mixed with herbs such as milk thistle and comfrey. Blue-green algae (see *Cyanobacteria*, pages 143–144) have been used in this way for the effective treatment of eczema. Clay (see page 130) and mud, including Dead Sea mud, are also excellent treatments when used in this manner. Therapeutic muds and mud peats impart a generous helping of bromine. Psoriatics can have lower than normal levels of this salt.

Rolled oats and oatmeal can also be used in packs and poultices, or merely slopped all over the skin.

PROGESTERONE CREAMS The application of cream containing the hormone progesterone has been found to be very effective for female psoriatics. A practitioner who treated menopause in patients who also happened to suffer with psoriasis reported impressive remissions when the cream was rubbed on psoriatic sites. Some sites which had been intractable for years cleared completely.[3] Common amongst such creams is the wild yam variety.

RHUBARB JUICE This contains anthraquinones (valuable agents in dyeing, evident in the brilliant bluish-red colour of the stalk and its flesh) which relieve itching and pain.

ROSEMARY More than a wonderful culinary herb and a sprig to indicate remembrance and fidelity. It is likely that you have used a shampoo or hair conditioner that contained rosemary oil. It has a valuable place in psoriasis treatment as an external stimulant and antiseptic. Add a sprig to hot bath water to create a therapeutic steam which can cleanse pores and stimulate circulation.

ROYAL JELLY Diluted with honey and water can be effective as a massage lubricant.

SARSAPARILLA TEA Applied topically has a calming effect.

SLIPPERY ELM POWDER Combined with a little pure water, this can be used as a soothing paste.

THYME This venerable herb contains the astringent tannin and the antiseptic thymol, which make it a valuable natural healing agent.

Scalp treatments
The scalp may also be oiled, using any of the natural cold-pressed oils listed above. This is best done at night before bed. A head wrap will avoid oil stains.

A very light lathering and a thorough rinsing in the morning will remove scaly particles lifted by the nightly regime. It will be required less frequently as improvement becomes obvious.

If your environmental bent allows it, take home a gallon container of seawater next time you're at the beach. Pour it over your head when you can allow it to remain for at least one hour, and to dry naturally.

Other topical treatments

Numerous proprietary brands of naturally derived or semi-natural surface preparations are available for the treatment of psoriasis. They invariably contain some good old standbys such as zinc oxide, essential oils or retinol (vitamin A). Many also contain an ingredient whose identity is not divulged by the maker because it is the factor which—alongside demonstrable success amongst their patients or clients—gives them the commercial edge. Whatever their ingredients, these products will only be of complete benefit when dietary and psychological factors are also addressed. Be warned that some might also contain a powerful steroid and therefore fall outside the essential criteria.

Capsaicin, a compound which blocks pain, and which is derived from chillies, is used to produce an ointment which is beneficial in the treatment of psoriasis.

The Pharbifarm range of products, developed by a former psoriatic and Scandinavian, is 100 per cent natural and completely drug-free. It contains mineral salts, four essential oils, and the 'secret' ingredient PS21 (a naturally derived plant extract). It has been used with success since the 1970s by psoriasis sufferers who persevere with the explicit directions, and without side-effects.

Bathing

Bathing is decidedly therapeutic when the bath water is enhanced with beneficial additives, of which a long list could be drawn. The addition of natural oils is an obvious consideration; the inclusion of half a cup of cold-pressed apple cider vinegar once a week will help neutralise the acid mantle.

One teaspoonful of tea-tree or bergamot oil in the bath once a week is also beneficial. Use bergamot at night or when the body will not be exposed to sunlight. The addition of oils such as lavender, bergamot or rosemary also provides valuable aromatherapy.

BRAN BATH This is created by suspending bran in a calico 'pillow' under a running tap or immersing it in the water; produces a milky, skin-softening soak. It is also effective in reducing itching. The bran can come from wheat, oats or rice, and the milk made from these can be added to the bath.

CLAY POWDER This can also be added to the bath. Not only do the French make the best cars, they also produce the best clay. Clay therapy has been used externally and internally, for cleansing and toning, for thousands of years (The Egyptians used it, and in *John* 9:11 in the Bible is the account of Jesus using clay to heal a blind man.) The clay used in pelotherapy is different from that which is used for pottery: in its structure, and in its composition of minerals and trace elements. Therapeutic clay has a high content of the powerful healing agent aluminium silica, in addition to rich deposits of calcium, copper, cobalt, magnesium, manganese, phosphorus, potassium and zinc. The clays suitable for healing are from the kaolinite, illite and smectite groups.

Each type of clay has slightly different properties, and its different level of mineral composition imbues the powder form with a characteristic colour. All clay suitable for healing has antiseptic and analgesic properties. Clay is extremely absorptive. It is also adsorptive, due to its magnetic properties, thus substances are drawn to the outside of the clay applied to the skin surface. In addition to removing toxins and cleaning the skin's pores, it will also stimulate the lymphatic system and blood circulation. It can be used in the bath, and in facial masks and poultices. Internal uses are described in the next chapter, *Internally—Nutrition for Skin Health*, see page 158.

Green clays are the most active and therefore the most widely used in medicine and cosmetics. Clays of other colours—yellow, red, pink and white—can also be purchased in powder form. Green clay is suitable for all skin types; its strongly astringent quality is especially good for oily skin and is the most effective for treating skin disorders. Yellow clay has similar drawing qualities to green clay. Red clay, while less absorbent, is suitable for dry and sensitive skin types. Pink clay is also good for sensitive and dehydrated skin. White clay, the mildest of all, is best for very sensitive and dry skin.

CHAMOMILE A wonderful herb with soothing properties when applied topically or taken as tea, it also adds a pleasing fragrance to the bath.

OATMEAL Has similar properties to chamomile and pleasing results.

TEA-TREE LAKES The effects of bathing in a tea-tree lake are also highly beneficial; this can be an amazing experience. This deeply dark water stained by the oil of tea-trees is very soft and the skin feels wonderfully supple and smooth after bathing in it.

Alternating hot and cold water showers of about two to three minutes each, and repeating this cycle several times before finishing with cold water, stimulate circulation.

Soaps

The Celts and Phoenicians used soap, the latter making it from goat tallow and wood ashes as early as 600 BC, for the treatment of skin conditions and as a hair gel. Synthetic detergents were developed by German chemists in 1916.[4]

Bath soaps, detergents, shampoos and conditioners can be anathema to sensitive skin. Depending on their type they may also harm non-sensitive skin. This is usually supposed to be because of fossil mineral and chemical ingredients. There is no soap that alone will heal skin afflictions.

Soap is a compound of fatty acid and an alkali. The alkali used is determined by the kind of soap being manufactured. Potash (potassium) is used for 'soft' soaps, while soda (sodium) is used for 'hard' soaps. The alkali imparts the better cleansing properties, and is present in considerable quantities in laundry soaps. Coconut and other vegetable oils are often used, but so are tallow, animal fats and alcohol. Glycerine and lanolin are used for their 'brilliance' (glycerine), and activity in overcoming the effect of excess free alkali (lanolin). Lanolin contains the same fats as the skin, together with cholesterol, sterols and the fatty acids. These are all emulsifying, protecting and penetrating.

The skin possesses an acid mantle, which means that in its balanced state it is acid, although the degree of acidity is constantly changing. It is most important to maintain the skin in an acid state. Alkaline soaps and detergents adversely affect even healthy skin and scalps, as in addition to removing dirt they remove the natural protective oils. It is very easy and common to overuse soap.

Olive oil is the principal ingredient in castile soap. This makes for a soap far superior to any which contain animal fats, for the latter can contribute to skin irritations. Olive or linseed oils are used with potassium and some alcohol in the manufacture of some surgical soaps.

Medicated soaps contain such substances as sulphur, terebene, salicylic acid, carbolic acid, corrosive sublimate (mercuric acid) and tar. A good grade of tar soap has been described as having a soothing effect on the skin. Give preference to wood tars (pine, beech), or juniper berry, and avoid the mineral-based coal tar.

When choosing a soap, avoid the medicated, perfumed and cheap varieties. Oatmeal soap, because of the grain ingredient, is beneficial to the circulation and peels off dead skin flakes. Castile and soaps composed of vegetable oils (almond and wheat germ, for example) and yoghurt soaps are recommended over any of the common consumer brands.

Shampoos

Psoriasis of the scalp can be the most tenacious of the disease's chosen sites. It is imperative to keep on top of this form (no pun intended), because if it is not at least treated topically it will return again and again and again. Our choice of shampoo is vital in these circumstances. Some people prefer the medicated varieties, but here the same principles apply as with our choice of soap. There is no harm in using castile soap as a shampoo. More particularly, a regular treatment with oils as described above could have a far more beneficial effect on the psoriatic scalp as a result of removing the dry plaque. We want a shampoo that imparts body and shine to our hair, and thereby promotes our self-esteem.

An excellent shampoo can be prepared at home with a few ingredients which will probably already have found a place in the bathroom cabinet, such as jojoba oil, rosemary oil, wheat germ oil and aloe vera. A pure shampoo base can be purchased from a health food store. A diluted apple cider vinegar rinse will leave the hair soft and shiny.

Sensitivity picture 1

It is taken as read that a person who has a skin ailment is temporarily disposed to sensitive skin. A number of factors should be considered when exposing the affected skin to the elements.

Water

Salt-water bathing is well known as being beneficial. A soak in the tub can be every bit as good. Be sure of your water supply, however. While the 'town supply' is chlorinated, fluoridated and processed to protect consumers from pollutants, it can be harsh on the skin. Applying a barrier cream or lotion such as lanolin before bathing or showering will provide protection.

Fresh air

Cell restoration is accomplished during sleep, when we breathe deeply and slowly. The quality of the air we breathe is fundamental to the level of our well-being.

Several decades ago, an autopsy performed in the Los Angeles morgue found the lungs of a non-smoker to be blackened and clogged. Pure air is essential to all humans if the skin is to function as it is designed. This applies equally to surrounding and inhaled air. Our air is not what it used to be prior to the Industrial Revolution. For that matter, nothing has been how it used to be since the introduction of fossil fuels as an energy source, but that's another story.

Overall, we should endeavour to get out of the hermetically sealed, fluorescent-lit and air conditioned capsule—read office/house/car—and breathe the stuff that keeps us alive. This, combined with some time in a pleasing space such as a forest, a garden, or anywhere outdoors away from an urban atmosphere, will also be a beneficial and vital respite from the artificial electromagnetism and radiation to which we are exposed in normal city living. Get off concrete and asphalt, and walk on the ground, on the grass or the sandy beach. This isn't some New Age guff—it's a simple fact. If you work all day with computers, you should go hug a tree occasionally, at least sit in a green space to re-orientate with the natural surroundings and breathe the air.

Sunlight

Sun baths—and therefore exposure to natural full-spectrum light—are essential. Calcium in the food (or supplementary) supply cannot be fully utilised without vitamin D. Exposure to natural full-spectrum light is the optimum source of natural vitamin D, which the body produces through the action of sunlight on the cholesterol that occurs naturally in the body. In this form, it is more readily utilised than artificial vitamin D in supplemental form. The pigmentation of darker-skinned people prevents most of the natural ultraviolet light from penetrating beneath the epidermis. Latitude and the amount of skin exposed to sunlight are also factors to consider, for sunlight is less intense the further away from the equator we live.

The sun's ultraviolet rays contain actinic rays that sterilise the skin. Sunbathing increases blood circulation. Overall, the stimulating effect of (safe, controlled) sunbathing is similar to exercise: general metabolism is improved, blood fats and cholesterol are reduced and blood viscosity is lessened, while oxygen levels are increased. Observe oiling before (with care if on a sandy beach) and especially afterwards.

Hormone production is improved by sunbathing. Melatonin is produced by the pineal gland when it is activated through the response of the retina of the eye to the ultraviolet light in sunlight. The production of other hormones by the lower brain and pituitary gland results from light entering the eye.

Natural full-spectrum light can increase taurine levels in the pituitary and pineal glands. A deficiency of natural light can result in taurine deficiency, which is a factor psoriatics should be aware of considering our special relationship with this amino acid which many of us have an inability to obtain via ordinary metabolism.

Excessive or prolonged exposure to the sun can result in skin cancer. Extreme sunspot activity increases the danger of over-exposure, particularly in the middle of the day. Sunbathing is best confined to early-to-mid-morning, or the period when the sun's rays impart their growing, healing qualities (named Kephra by the Egyptians).

'Diet' soft drinks—which all contain artificial sweeteners, which are excitotoxins—drunk while sunbathing have been known to cause dark, permanent blotches on the skin.[5]

Clothing

The skin deserves to be in the presence of natural fibres. Synthetic clothing restricts the body's ability to breathe and robs it of vital energy.

Sensitivity picture 2

Photosensitivity

Any person can be sensitive to the results of exposure to sunlight in the presence of a sensitising agent or phototoxin such as a furocoumarin. Phototoxicity can result from the combination of a phototoxic agent and exposure to sunlight in those who are photosensitive. Typical responses are tingling, burning, itching and a general redness and swelling. The reaction is limited to the sun-exposed parts, and it will develop any time from between a few minutes and several hours after sun exposure. The response may be only temporary, depending upon the discontinued use of the phototoxin, but sometimes permanent blotching can result. Photosensitisers are highly photosensitive chemical agents which have been found to contain phototoxins and photoallergens. They occur in a long list of consumer items and widely prescribed treatments, including deodorant soaps, which contain halogenated salicylanides.[6]

Oil of bergamot

Bergamot is a very useful herb, but in some people who are photosensitive the oil can cause berlock dermatitis, a topical reaction that can result in permanent dark irritating blotches. In its earliest stages berlock dermatitis manifests as rashes and blistering burns.

Oil of rosemary and oil of lavender, which with oil of bergamot are common ingredients in many perfumes, can produce similar reactions under sun exposure.

People who take drinks laced with artificial sweeteners—aspartame, saccharin—while sunbathing lay themselves open to photosensitive reactions. Lime juice or lime essence, ingredients common in many shaving creams, after-shaves, soft drinks and some perfumes, can also produce photoallergenic reactions in those who are susceptible. These can be very toxic for some people due to their furocoumarin content.

Furocoumarins

These are chemicals (polyphenols) which occur naturally in some foods and herbs, namely lemons, limes, bergamot, celery, carrots, parsnips, parsley, figs, dill and fennel. PUVA therapy employs a furocoumarin (psoralen). (See also *Antioxidants*, pages 164–166)

Photobiology

Light and colour therapy have been used to treat a variety of diseases and can be worth exploring as adjuncts to dealing with our psoriatic state. Different colours in the spectrum can exert various influences on the personality and senses. This knowledge is used in disciplines as far apart as marketing and health services. For example, cool colours have been used to sell menthol cigarettes and red is used in restaurants to stimulate appetite; pink has been used in rehabilitation centres because of its soothing effect, although this was found to decline after prolonged use with the same subjects. Local councils and municipalities employ colour to influence 'behavioural problems'. For example, 'passive pink' has been experimented with in attempts to deter graffitists, and at one time London's Blackfriars Bridge was repainted blue in an attempt to reduce the number of suicides from it.

Colours have been experimentally shown to affect health. Different colours can affect blood pressure, pulse and respiration rates, brain activity and biorhythms. In some postnatal wards in the 1970s, blue lights were used to replace blood transfusions for premature babies born with potentially fatal neonatal jaundice. In the same wards, gold light was used to soothe hospital staff irritated by the blue light. In the same decade, coal miners in the (then) Soviet Union were showered with ultraviolet light as a preventative measure against black lung disease. Ultraviolet light has also been used in Russian schoolrooms to supplement harsh white fluorescent light, with perceived results which included faster growth and work rates, improved grades and lower incidences of catarrhal infections. In the United States fluorescent light has been used in conjunction with psoralens to treat herpes. (See also *Colour Therapy,* page 190.)

7 Internally—nutrition for skin health

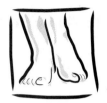

... to attack the skin problem cosmetically does not get to the cause. The first thing to think about when attacking a skin problem is to understand that the skin is one way for the body to release toxins. Thus there is a fair chance that the body is overloaded with toxins in this case.

Helping to clear the alimentary system is one thing to keep in mind. Also helping the liver to clear the blood is another. Helping the kidneys work is still another. Thus these three areas must be the focal points of attack for most skin problems.

In addition to helping the body to release toxins, one must do whatever is possible to reduce the intake of toxins ... And finally, there is need to provide all essential nutrients to normalise the metabolism of the body. This simply means to make the body work as it should.

Maurice Finkel [1]

You are unique

While psoriatics have many things in common, we must each identify the appropriate individual approach to and management of our own dietary and treatment program. Again, our best help will come from a talented and knowledgeable nutritionist. This is because of the vital role which diet (in combination with other forms of treatment) can play in gaining the upper hand with skin disease.

Optimum nutrition is not only gaining the greatest value from the foods we ingest, and therefore promoting full and complete metabolism, it is also understanding our individual metabolic needs, and accepting and understanding that one-size-fits-all diets are irrelevant.

In 1956, Dr Roger Williams, who is credited with discovering vitamin B5 (pantothenic acid), coined the principle of biochemical individuality. In his book of the same name, Dr Williams points out that our organs are of different shapes and sizes and that, furthermore, our bodies have different levels of enzymes and individual metabolic patterns and rates of digestion. We have different determined nutrient needs that are of genetic origin (some people need more folic acid than others, for instance). Each of us has a need for a different daily allowance of vitamins, minerals and proteins.

Our genetic, racial and environmental heritages all have a role to play in what is required by and of our bodies in their relationship with good nutrition. An exclusively macrobiotic diet is probably not all that pertinent for a cattleman in Missouri.

The practice of identifying and applying individual nutritional needs is labelled 'metabolic typing'. Under this system essentially we are classed as one of two main types, with an intermediate type overlapping and sharing characteristics of the first two. The three types are named slow oxidisers, fast oxidisers and mixed oxidisers.

Oxidation is the provision of glucose (energy) to cells; slow, fast and mixed oxidation underpin how our body deals with proteins, fats and carbohydrates, and consequently indicates our need for them in our daily diet. A slow oxidiser requires a low-protein, low-fat, high-carbohydrate diet; fast oxidisers require high-protein, high-fat, low-carbohydrate diets. A mixed oxidiser requires relatively equal amounts of each nutrient. According to the principles of metabolic typing, if one's genetic need is not met by these nutrients being made available in the required proportions for proper utilisation, when they are needed, inefficiency at the cellular level will result, organ function will be weakened, the body system will become stressed and ultimately damage will be caused through imbalance in the whole body system.

Vital factors for skin health

Diets for skin health

Because each of us is unique the optimum quantity of any single nutrient differs from person to person, influenced by factors such as genetic indisposition, circumstances and the nature of a diseased state. Thus your particular requirements for nutrient factors, or combinations of factors, differ from mine.

Supplementation with amino acids, for example, should be guided by a professional practitioner, because they need to be added to the diet in combination with the nutrients with which they are normally associated in the metabolic process, to ensure against toxicity and nutrient imbalance. This stipulation applies to the use of any nutrient, be it a vitamin, mineral or essential fatty acid. (The principal minerals for psoriatics are calcium, magnesium, silicon and chlorine.)

The average digestive system contains 7 pounds (3 kilograms) of mostly friendly (probiotic) bacteria, which promote the production of digestive enzymes and the body's ability to deal effectively with unfriendly bacteria. The Western diet, antibiotics, stress and pollution can be detrimental to the friendly bacteria. Cultured foods provide the probiotics *Lactobacillus acidophilus*, *Bifidobacteria* and *Casei* which can be very beneficial to the variety of intestinal disorders which affect a large proportion of psoriatics. It is questionable, however, whether their prime sources—yoghurts and fermented milk drinks—are ideal for the psoriatic. Probiotics are available in supplement form.

Rejuvenation

It is important to begin a nutritional program with a strong and clean foundation. If you were to attend a natural health clinic, a controlled fast will likely figure prominently in the initial phases of treatment, because the necessary first step in arresting decline is detoxification. A properly controlled fast will also give the digestive system a rest. Colonic irrigation might be another worthwhile avenue to pursue.

Fasting is a perfectly natural process. The body has inbuilt self-cleansing mechanisms and is also capable of accommodating fasting. During a fast, the body will draw its nourishment from its own reserves, from tissue and other sources including the toxins that are being eliminated. The fat stores will be the first to be called upon, and fluids the first to be eliminated. Other tissues will only be called upon when all fat residue is exhausted, and the vital organs all can afford to give over safe and limited quantities of their own substances to sustain the normal condition of heart, brain and blood.

It is essential to seek the assistance of an experienced and qualified person to help you plan and work through an appropriate level of fasting.

If fasting is out for you—and certain types should not fast at all, notably diabetics and people with heart and kidney problems—consider eating less as a general rule. Leaner people live longer.

Some foods for healing (A–Z)

Naturally, fresh vegetables and fruits are highest on the list of essential foods for the psoriatic. Ideally they will be organic. Community food co-operatives are a very good source of high quality organic produce and most of the other products on the shopping list of the serious self-healer. Many regular fruit and vegetable outlets also sell organic fresh produce these days. Co-operatives and centres like them (e.g. health food stores) are also a worthy source of additional information on nutrition. In the case of co-operatives, the (usually) higher cost of the organic produce can be offset by membership and active participation in the running of the business. Such participation can also be beneficial to the overall healing process. You could also consider growing your own organic produce. In fact alfalfa, the first plant in the following list, is one which provides the opportunity to start with, in its sprouted form.

ALFALFA From the Arabic for (approximately) 'father of all foods', alfalfa is a rich source of minerals, vitamins A, B, D, E and K, and protein. It is very common in the modern Western diet in its sprouted form, and rightly so because of the eight enzymes it provides, which are essential to gut action and proper nutrient assimilation. A strong antifungal, it is also thought to be effective in reducing cholesterol.

ALOE VERA An enzyme-rich digestive aid and cell rejuvenator. It is widely acclaimed for its revivifying, detoxifying and proteolytic qualities, and as an immune system ally. The aloe genus, part of the Lily family, offers 275 different species. It is the species *Aloe vera* that is considered the most beneficial in terms of its medicinal qualities. Aloe vera juice contains more than 100 vitamins, minerals, enzymes and plant compounds that are essential for cell growth and renewal. Taken as a juice, aloe vera stimulates the growth of skin cells, acts enzymatically to digest and dissolve damaged or dead tissue cells, and promotes blood cleansing. Topical application of the juice or pulp relieves itching.

The plant has been used for thousands of years as a topical treatment. When taken internally, the ingredients act as powerful detoxifying agents that improve tissue function in a synergistic relationship with the body's immune system. The juice makes available an abundance of mucopolysaccharides (long-chain sugars which are the body's building blocks). The young body is capable of manufacturing these itself, but this replication ceases at about age ten. Things change, the body concentrates on becoming a sexual being and relies on outside sources of these building blocks. Aloe vera is one of the richest plant sources.

Intestinal permeability can arise from a lack of mucopolysaccharides. Their replenishment through the ingestion of aloe vera juice could do wonders for many psoriatics.

AVOCADOS These delicious fruits have been given the seal of approval by leading orthodox health researchers and the National Heart Foundation of Australia. A study at the Wesley Medical Centre in Brisbane, Australia, found that eating a half or whole avocado a day had a direct relationship with weight loss and reduced cholesterol levels.[2]

CELERY SEED Promotes a healthy circulatory system. Celery seed preparations are used in prescriptive products for rheumatoid arthritis.

CEREAL GRAINS Here I am referring to whole grains. Bread is the staff of life—but is it? Perhaps this depends on the type and quality of bread. The patriarch of a bread-making dynasty once allowed a slip in a discussion with a journalist. When asked if he enjoyed the company's most popular sliced refined white loaf, he responded, 'Certainly not! I wouldn't eat the stuff.' He further remarked that he preferred wholegrain bread.[3]

The quality of bread as a food is greatly influenced by the manner of its making, and of course by the quality of the grains used. In addition to gluten, preservatives and other additives, the ubiquitous white loaf is made with flour that is almost pure starch. The introduction of steel roller mills in flour milling processes in the late eighteenth century, first in Hungary and soon afterwards in Britain, largely sounded the death knell for the goodness that is in the grain. High-speed roller-milling destroys whatever of the fragile germ remains from the sifting and processing. It is vital to the flour-milling industry's profits that the flour that is produced has a long shelf life. Wheat germ does not, for it quickly becomes rancid and spoils the rest of the flour. The white stuff is the wrong stuff for anyone who is serious about eating good food. Opt for organic stoneground flours and breads that are made with the whole grain. Sourdough, and breads that are naturally leavened and contain no sugar, no salt and no preservatives, are readily available and infinitely superior to those that cannot claim these benefits. A sourdough bakery is likely to be operated by individuals who pursue sound ecological practices, and therefore will not be using unwanted additives and excitotoxins in their doughs and pastries.

A substance in wheat bran called phytate, which can inhibit the absorption of some essential minerals, is broken down by baker's yeast. Note that phytate remains unaltered in unleavened bread, chapattis, soda bread, breakfast cereal to which bran is added, and other bran products.

Consider also the gluten factor in grains. Gluten is present in wheat, oats, barley and rye. Corn and buckwheat are okay, as are the gluten-free flours produced from millet, rice, tapioca and potato.

CHLOROPHYLL An excellent blood purifier, blood builder and promoter of circulation, which is absorbed readily via cell membranes in the mouth, stomach and intestines. Commercially produced from alfalfa concentrate or *Chlorella*, a marvellous freshwater alga, liquid chlorophyll is a natural alkaline internal cleanser and tonic.

Chlorophyll's ready absorption and affinity with the blood supply arises from its molecular similarity to human blood. Human haemoglobin and chlorophyll share almost identical molecular structures, the pyrrole rings, with the only difference between the two being that chlorophyll has a magnesium ion at its molecular core while iron is at the centre of the human blood molecule. Magnesium imparts the green colour to chlorophyll while iron imparts red to the blood.

In addition to being present in large amounts in spirulina and AFA (see *Cyanobacteria* below), chlorophyll is obtained from green vegetables of course, and also sea vegetables, wheat grass and barley grass. It is easily ingested in its liquid form. *Chlorella* is the richest known source of chlorophyll, containing 50 times the level in alfalfa.

Chlorophyll makes for an excellent mouthwash and deodoriser, and can also be added to juice drinks, soups, stews, and salad dressing.

CULTURED FOODS These are both pre-digested and enzyme-providing. Amongst them miso, the paste made from fermented soybeans and grain, and sourdough leavened bread can be worthy additions to the psoriatic's pantry— the first as a flavoursome additive to soups and as an alternative spread on the second.

CYANOBACTERIA This is perhaps not an overly inviting name for a food, and for that matter nor is its common name, blue-green algae. This is the staple food of most aquatic creatures, ranging from the microscopic organisms in lakes to the whale, and is related to plankton, seaweed and kelp. It is comprised of simple monocellular organisms and is a rich source of amino acids, minerals, trace elements and enzymes. (See *Tables* in *Appendix 1*.) Low in calories and with zero cholesterol, cyanobacteria provides more calcium than milk, more protein than meat, and essential fatty acids. Importantly for the vegetarian, both forms provide the essential amino acids methionine and phenylalanine which are otherwise only available in animal meat and dairy products. This is especially significant given the psoriatic's need for methionine.

These algae stimulate friendly bacteria growth in the intestines. They are a great ally of the immune system through the antioxidant pigments present in chlorophyll and beta-carotene, and highly effective in stimulating the macrophages, and hence T cells and NK cells, thus revitalising the liver, spleen, thymus, adenoids, lymph nodes and bone marrow. These organs and constituents are then better able to manage stress caused by toxic invasion or a disease state. Cyanobacteria can also be applied as a beneficial surface treatment.

This nutritious green plant food should not be confused with ordinary pond bacteria. It is commercially farmed. The two principal types of freshwater cultivated and wild cyanobacteria are spirulina (*Spirulina platensis*) and AFA (*Afanzomenon flos-aquae*). It is a natural food source, available as a supplement, and highly complementary to the average Western diet. Wild AFA is 95 per cent assimilable, and is believed to be better for its beneficial effect on the mind and emotions than spirulina, which is 80 to 90 per cent assimilable and more beneficial for body nourishing and building.

Another freshwater alga, *Chlorella*, was the largest-selling health food in Japan in the mid-1990s. It contains approximately 60 per cent protein (including all the essential amino acids) compared with the soybean's 30 per cent.

As with many of the food and dietary alternatives presented here, for many people a change of attitude will probably be necessary to accept that this or that substance could be beneficial to them in the first instance, and in the second to actually bring themselves to try it out. It is entirely understandable that someone who has been raised on the notion that animal meats are the only worthwhile source of protein would greet the suggestion that they ingest whale fodder with anything less than derision. Often it requires a severe health crisis to bring one to this decisive point.

FIBRE With the news that fibre was essential in the diet, a whole generation lurched into eating wheat bran and opting for wholegrain 'bran-enriched' breads over the ubiquitous processed white loaf.

Soluble dietary fibres are gel-like substances that absorb water in the intestines. Roughage (fibre) is essential in the diet, and is easily obtained from fresh raw fruits and vegetables. The fibres present in the skins of fruits and vegetables are largely indigestible. This is important in dietary fibre's role, if you recall that principal amongst its functions is to help maintain the tone of the intestinal wall, and to ease the progress of proper elimination—it is a silent partner in the digestive process with very little of it being digested and absorbed. The exception is hemicellulose, which is digested by bacteria in the colon.

Whole grains provide a good source of fibre, with oat bran highest on the list and wheat bran lowest, owing to its high cellulose content, which is adverse to the management of cholesterol. Apples—specifically their fibre pectin—are a very worthwhile source.

FRUITS Virtually all fruits (with the exception of citrus for most psoriatics) are essential in any diet and provide not only obvious nutrients but also micronutrients which aid in their digestion. Opt for organically grown fruit for preference, and eat those skins which are edible—first thoroughly washing the fruit.

GAMMA-LINOLENIC ACIDS (GLAs) These are members of the group of essential fatty acids, and in turn are comprised of linoleic (omega-6) and alpha-linolenic (omega-3) fatty acids. They are the originating site for the production of the hormone-like prostaglandins. These compounds stimulate and control various functions such as keeping the blood thin, improving nerve and immune function, and maintaining the body's water balance. Psoriatics are generally deficient in GLAs, and both omega-6 and omega-3 are known to be beneficial in arthritis treatment.

Approximately 60 per cent of the brain and nervous system consists of fatty acids. We synthesise less GLAs as we grow older, and supplementation can become necessary.

The omega-6 family of fats is derived exclusively from seeds and their oils, of which hemp, evening primrose and borage are the best known sources. Sunflower, safflower, sesame and wheat germ oil are also fine sources. The omega-3 family is similarly provided in linseed and pumpkin seed oils, and fish oil. Indeed, linseed oil is the richest known source of alpha-linolenic acid.

Only those individuals on an extremely rigid no-fat diet are likely to be deficient in omega-6. Nevertheless, supplementary intake is available from good natural sources such as evening primrose oil, sunflower, safflower and corn oils.

Omega-3 and omega-6 should be taken in combination to meet the essential requirements of a balanced intake. When only one is taken, a deficiency of the other could result.

GRAPE SEED EXTRACT Extracts of grape seed and grapefruit strengthen blood vessel walls and reduce inflammation. They stabilise collagen and elastin, and can improve connective tissue health. In addition to being a powerful antifungal agent, grape seed extract is also a natural antihistamine, antiviral and antibacterial. As an antioxidant, grape seed extract has been found to be more effective than vitamins C and E. These extracts are taken as drops in fluid—they are very bitter and require some assimilation with the tastebuds at first.

GREEN BARLEY This is a superb blood purifier which provides chlorophyll, vitamins and minerals, and is effective in helping to build strong, healthy blood cells, in particular neutrophils, the primary blood cleansers.

HERBS Herbal preparations, in the form of teas, extracts or tinctures, or in a pure cream or lotion, can be useful for both alleviating skin surface discomfort and addressing overactive cell division and internal problems associated with psoriasis. Culinary herbs such as anise, basil and coriander can also be powerful digestive aids. Recourse to specific literature and the input of a talented herbalist are essential to gain the greatest benefit from the use of herbs.[4] (See also *Table 5* in *Appendix 1*.)

A worthwhile tea can be infused from a blend of burdock, mistletoe, motherwort, passionflower and wild lettuce.

Anise One of numerous digestive aids, recognised by its aniseed flavour.

American yellow saffron Highlighted by Edgar Cayce as beneficial to the treatment of permeable intestine. He recommended its use in the evening, with a pinch of slippery elm bark (see page 148) in the morning.

Barberry The bark of the herb's root is an excellent natural source of the beneficial alkaloid berberine. The berries are also therapeutic. Berberine is effective in inhibiting the excessive skin cell regeneration, and promotes the secretion of bile which makes it invaluable to liver function and general digestive health.

Basil A culinary herb and immune system stimulant.

Cat's claw Contains alkaloids of the friendly variety, which provide its immune-boosting qualities. Do not combine with vaccines, hormones or medical immunotherapies. Not suitable for children or when pregnant.

Chamomile An immune stimulator. Widely used as a pre-bedtime tea and a natural source of calcium.

Comfrey To give it its proper due, comfrey is used successfully in topically treating skin ulceration and tissue damage, including the results of severe burns, and varicose ulcers, and internally in the treatment of bronchial and chest infections, gastric ulcers and general digestive health, and female disorders. Home gardeners also appreciate comfrey's powerful contribution to the compost heap both as a superb source of calcium and other minerals, and in its effect in breaking down the heap more rapidly.

Despite its hairy, somewhat prickly leaves, comfrey can be a beneficial additive to salads or even munched solo. Whether eaten raw or infused as a tea (or in topical treatments), this herb is one of the few vegetable sources of B_{12}, is a rich source of vitamins A and C, calcium, potassium, phosphorus and other trace minerals, and provides some protein. Comfrey also provides vitamins B_1, B_2, D, E, niacin, pantothenic acid and choline. It is a valued cleanser and can promote circulation. Vegetarians do well to include comfrey in the diet to provide the amino acid lysine.

This is also a vital plant for the psoriatic because it contains allantoin and therefore, in addition to its beneficial action on damaged skin, this herb when used internally helps heal intestinal irritability and is generally of remedial assistance in the presence of digestive disorders.

Caution: Severe liver damage has been caused by the pyrrolizidine alkaloids which are present in the comfrey root. People with liver disease and alcoholics should not use comfrey, and it should not be provided in dietary form to children under two years of age. Some comfrey preparations for internal application that are pyrrolizidine alkaloid-free are available.

Dandelion An antioxidant, useful in treating liver and kidney disorders, and assists with calming inflammation of the bowel. Dandelion increases activity of the pancreas and liver, and aids the digestion of fats. The root, roasted and ground, makes an excellent alternative to coffee and tea.

Goldenseal A useful antibacterial agent. Eminently versatile, it is used in unguents, and also with great effect in promoting a healthy digestive system. It is the particular alkaloids which goldenseal contains which are helpful in treating problematic mucous membranes. It increases bile and gastric juice secretion, and is useful for toning the liver. Goldenseal also contains berberine.

Milk thistle This herb contains silymarin, which is a flavenoid antioxidant, an anti-inflammatory, immune-enhancing free radical scavenger more powerful than vitamin E, and a combination of three active ingredients (flavenolignans) called silybin, silychristin and silydianin. These compounds support immune modulation, stabilise and help develop healthy new liver cells, and can arrest alcohol damage to the liver. Silymarin also changes the construction of liver cells' membrane, provides protection against invading toxins, and deals with those that do manage to infiltrate the organ. It is also effective against poisonous fungi, and is an antidote against leukotriene B4 which is implicated in psoriasis.

Milk thistle supports healthy liver growth and maintenance even in the face of alcohol malpractice. This could be the 'milk drink' for the youth about to embark on a night on the town who downs a pint of milk to give the stomach 'a lining'. Silymarin can reverse liver damage and toxicity from alcohol, drugs and pollutants. Milk thistle normalises the liver's ability to produce cholesterol and other phospholipids. At the very least, milk thistle will improve enzyme levels to deal with liver and gall bladder action that is sluggish in the presence of fatty and oily foods.

Milk thistle products are sold in dried and powdered seed forms, tablets, capsules and fluid extracts. Follow directions to avoid over-activating the liver.

Red clover A phytoestrogen rich in isoflavones and therefore beneficial for its antioxidant properties, this herb has been used for a variety of medicinal purposes in far-flung corners where it is a native crop, including Australia. It has also been used by generations of farmers as a soil improver, due to its nitrogen-fixing qualities, and is one of the world's oldest agricultural crops, a valuable source of hay for livestock and nectar for bees.

Rosemary Amongst this herb's active ingredients is borneol, an oil compound which stimulates the secretion of saliva and digestive juices and helps maintain an efficient digestive tract. Rosemary also inspires liver action, and will generally improve blood circulation. Herbalists also know its value as a tonic that soothes the nervous system while sharpening brain power. In addition to the fresh herb, rosemary is available as an essential oil.

Caution Follow the directions for the oil's use carefully and do not ingest it without the advice and direction of a practitioner.

Sarsaparilla Contains sarsaponin (saponins, a fibrous compound which is also present in ginseng, soybeans, chick peas, lentils, peanuts, mung, kidney and broad beans, asparagus, oats and spinach), a powerful blood purifier, immune system stimulant and antidote against the toxic effects of poisons. Sarsaponin binds with endotoxins that are implicated in psoriasis. It also binds with and expels bile salts and sterols, and thus has a role in reducing cholesterol levels. The sarsaparilla plant's root provides the hormones testosterone and progesterone, and cortin, one of the adrenal hormones.

Slippery elm This is actually slippery elm bark, obtained from the inner bark of the mature elm tree (*Ulmus fulva*), native to and widespread throughout North America and a relative of the mighty European elm. Effective against inflammatory irritations and identified by Edgar Cayce as a valuable agent in the treatment of intestinal permeability. The mucilage and cereal starch in slippery elm are also effective in separating protein particles from cow's milk, which makes it easier to digest.

The tragedy inherent in the use of slippery elm is that commercial methods of stripping the bark can disfigure or kill the tree. Given that Native North Americans used the bark as a medicine and natural food preservative throughout their long history, it is possible to harvest it without causing this damage. Always examine the label to determine whether the powder was produced by natural, sustainable methods.

JUICES Fruit and vegetable juices are an excellent source of nutrition and vitalising, dehydration-countering liquid. The juices of strawberries, cherries and celery also aid the excretion of uric acid. Freshly squeezed fruit juice is best first thing in the morning, as the fructose it contains provides a fine, quick, energising wake-up drink. Fruits and vegetables lend themselves to some wonderful juice combinations. Apple, beetroot, blackcurrant, carrot, celery, comfrey, parsley and wheat grass juices are good for the psoriatic.

KELP A wonder food, which with many other sea vegetables (see pages 153–154) is antibacterial and antiviral, in addition to being highly alkaline and a rich mineral source. It sustains the health of mucous membrane and can lower cholesterol levels and blood pressure. Kelp powder and granules can be used in many ways, as a seasoning ingredient in soups and sauces, and simply sprinkled over food. Individuals who are diagnosed with thyroid conditions should consult for direction with using kelp products because of their high iodine content.

LECITHIN A member of the phospholipid class of fats, lecithin is a body and brain food, renowned for its work against excess cholesterol and fats. It increases immunity, cleanses the liver and promotes a healthy nervous system. It is high in choline, which is an important co-enzyme in metabolism and a chemical detoxifier. Lecithin was discovered in egg yolk in 1850 by the French researcher Maurice Gobley. Named from the Greek *lekthos* (egg yolk), lecithin today is produced mostly from soybeans and is widely used as an emulsifier in food products. Lecithin is composed of phospholipids, phosphoric acid, choline and inositol, and methionine. The liver produces lecithin constantly, for it is an essential constituent in bile production. It is also produced by cholesterol. Lecithin's good work is done on the lipid particles in circulation; its emulsification of these reduces their size, which helps to keep the blood clear. The solubility of cholesterol in bile is dependent on the presence of lecithin, and even more so on the presence of the correct proportions of lecithin, cholesterol and bile salts. Lecithin's ability to quickly convert body fats into energy makes it a beneficial adjunct to the treatment of skin disorders.

Lecithin is also a valuable brain food, as it improves memory. Thirty per cent of the dry weight of the brain is lecithin. One of its major ingredients, choline, in itself plays an important role in balanced physical and emotional behaviour. Choline synthesises in the body to form acetylcholine, a deficiency of which can adversely affect brain function. Such deficiencies can increase with age thus, in conjunction with its positive effects on fat metabolism, the addition of lecithin to a daily regime in the case of older psoriatics could offer a multiplicity of beneficial effects.

In addition to its presence in every cell, lecithin is also obtained from foods such as sardines and anchovies, liver, nuts, egg yolk, soybeans and whole wheat. It is also available as a food supplement in the form of liquid, granules and capsules.

Cooking destroys lecithin. Natural butter contains both lecithin and cholesterol, which is a proper combination. In pasteurised butter, the lecithin has been destroyed and only cholesterol is left.

LENTILS, PULSES AND BEANS These provide alternatives to the conventional diet's sources of protein, vitamins and essential minerals. They straddle the alkaline-acid food balance. Green and brown lentils provide selenium, iron, manganese, phosphorus, and vitamins B1 and B6. Raw lentils and chick peas contain trypsin inhibitors, which prevent protein from being completely digested. This is overcome when they are cooked or sprouted.

Popular members of the group include aduki beans, black-eye beans, brown, red and green lentils, mung beans, pinto beans, red kidney beans and split peas.

Pulses are high in purines, which should be avoided by people who suffer from gout. (See also *Table 6* in *Appendix 1*.)

LINSEED (FLAXSEED) Known for millennia for its healing properties, the oil obtained from this seed increases the metabolic rate and improves immune functioning. The seed's content of lignans (phytoestrogens) is especially beneficial for female psoriatics. In addition to being effective in treatment of pre-menstrual tension, the lignans are antiviral and antifungal. Eating the seed or consuming the oil will stimulate the intestinal bacteria to produce up to 800 times more of the lignans than is produced by the consumption of any other food.[5]

Linseed oil is the richest known source of unsaturated alpha-linolenic acid, which is one of the omega-3 fatty acids so essential in the skin-repairing diet. The seed meal or oil provides phospholipids, including lecithin, and therefore emulsifies fats and oils in the body. Valuable levels of vitamin E and carotene are also provided.

MAGNESIUM-CONTAINING FOODS These foods are alkaline and take up the acid in the system, converting it to neutral salts. Such foods stimulate peristalsis and bowel action, and promote fat assimilation. See *Appendix 1* for natural sources, of which molasses is one.

MOLASSES An extremely rich source of calcium and iron, vitamin E and the B vitamins, including pantothenic acid, plus inositol, copper, magnesium and phosphorus. Molasses is a residue of (both cane and beet) sugar production.

OLIVES—FRUIT, OIL, LEAF AND BARK EXTRACTS Olive oil increases bile secretion and encourages peristalsis. It is said that olive oil dissolves cholesterol and soothes the mucous membranes.

PAPAYA (PAWPAW) This wonderful fruit has a very high vitamin A content, provides high levels of calcium, magnesium and potassium, and is a good source of vitamin C. It is also an excellent source of the amino acids leucine, lysine, methionine, phenylalanine, threonine, tryptophan and valine. The pepsin in papaya works effectively on protein and some starch digestion, making it an important digestive food.

RAW FOODS A diet which is solely or predominantly based on raw food is ideal for the psoriatic and will provide great relief to the liver. Try shredding, grinding, juicing, pureeing and liquefying.

The Bircher-Benner Clinic in Zurich, Switzerland, is quite explicit in its directions on the requirement and efficacy of a specialised, individually determined raw vegetarian food diet in the early stages of psoriasis treatment. This clinic leads the field in the natural treatment of skin disease, and its co-founder is the originator of Bircher muesli. Dr Vogel, another Swiss physician with excellent credentials, also stresses the importance of a raw food diet. In the considered opinion of the Bircher-Benner clinic, a raw food diet which also excludes fat should be maintained for up to three months. It is particularly important when obesity accompanies the skin condition.

The withdrawal of salt is also stated as being very important to this dietary program, particularly when kidney malfunctions are also evident. The clinic is specific in its withdrawal of not only salt itself, but also foods that are rich in sodium. By retaining fluid in tissues, this mineral causes swelling and susceptibility to secondary skin complaints. Foods with a high sodium content (which would be best avoided in the psoriatic diet anyway) include clams, crab, shrimps, cheese, brains, liver, ham, and poultry. MSG is also high in sodium.

The benefit of raw foods over cooked foods, in any diet, has much to do with the nature of the enzymes present in them. They are 'weaker' than the body's digestive juices and when consumed stimulate the secretion of weaker hydrochloric acid. This has the effect of enabling greater and more enduring performance of particular enzymes in the food. This process also places a lesser load on the pancreas and liver. Indeed, the pancreas can become enlarged through the regular or continuous consumption of cooked food.

Cooking destroys the natural enzymes in fresh food when the temperature reaches only 118°F (48°C). True, they are going to be destroyed during digestion anyway, but sufficient enzymes survive the onslaught of stomach acid to allow their absorption via the intestine. Food temperature is important overall, because digestion in the stomach proceeds only when the food reaches body temperature. Very cold foods thus pose an obvious problem for the digestive system.

Ultimately, however, the freshness of food is the intrinsic factor in obtaining optimum nutrients. Even where fresh fruits and vegetables are organically grown, their goodness is dissipated within hours of having been picked. This is because the plant lipids called sterols and sterolins are vital for only six to eight hours after harvesting. Cooking further destroys what small level of plant lipids survives after transportation to market and storage on the shelf.

RICE This is possibly the best grain for the psoriatic because it is the least allergenic of the grains. Organic brown rice provides most of the vitamin B complex and valuable minerals. Unlike white rice, brown rice possesses gamma oryzanol, an antioxidant and antifungal substance. It is easy to digest.

The whole grain variety is infinitely superior to the polished variety, and only the organically grown form should be purchased. This is not only because of the over-reliance of sprays in growing the non-organic crop, but also because of the use of contaminants to 'protect' stored grains for long periods of time, and their absence in certified organic varieties.

Rice bran improves the function of the intestinal wall and achieves a balance in bowel bacteria. In this it is more effective than wheat bran. The latter contains insoluble fibre, whereas the bran in rice is soluble.

ROYAL JELLY This is the highest natural source of pantothenic acid. This vitamin (B5) can improve the body's ability to deal with stress, aids the adrenal gland in maintaining a proper blood sugar level, and promotes energy and stamina. It greatly revitalises the endocrine system.

Royal jelly is an easy-to-digest source of concentrated nutrients. In addition to B5 it provides folic acid, amino acids, fatty acids and carbohydrates, and zinc, sulphur, sodium, potassium, iron, and traces of chromium, manganese and nickel.

Caution People with allergies should not use royal jelly.

SALTS AND SEASONINGS While commercial table salt is a good source of iodine, there are better sources. Rock salt and sea salt are in a less processed and refined state. Vegetable salt is also a rich source and provides additional flavours. Gomashio is a delicious and nutritious table salt which is made by combining lightly roasted sesame seeds and sea salt in a ratio of 5:1, and pounding in a mortar and pestle or food processor. (See also *Alternatives*, pages 168–172.)

SEA VEGETABLES Kelp and edible sea grasses provide vitamins (including high levels of B_{12}), minerals (at many times the values present in land vegetables) and protein (providing a wide range of amino acids). They are generally antibacterial, antiviral and antifungal, and effective in promoting the health of mucous membranes. Some sea vegetables provide more calcium than any other food, and many times the iron of spinach and egg yolks. Seaweed extract can increase bifidobacteria levels in the intestine.

The regular inclusion of sea vegetables in the diet can effectively reduce the levels of cholesterol and other fats in the blood, and generally aid digestion. This is largely due to the plant sterol beta-sitosterol, present in sea vegetables, which is an effective agent in lowering cholesterol.

There are various types of edible seaweeds, and the names by which they are generally known and marketed in their dried state derive from the Japanese. Their addition to a meal can lend a whole new dynamic to the eating and nutritional experience, a secret that has been understood for centuries by civilisations including the Japanese.

Kelp tablets are produced from the rockweeds; Irish moss is the source of carrageen (the gelatinous vegetable gum) which is used in cosmetics and some pharmaceuticals, and in food processing. It is one substance used in food processing which has some beneficial or worthwhile presence. Algin, from giant brown kelp, is also used as an emulsifier in food production.

Organic gardeners are well-versed in the huge benefits of seaweed extracts in their labours, and mainstream farmers have been onto the beneficial uses of sea-vegetable products for soil treatment and stock feeds for decades.

Agar-agar A clear, glutinous vegetable used for thickening in any dish, sweet or savoury, as an alternative to gelatine and gluten sources. It is a powerful antioxidant, and as a digestive aid its fibre quality assists peristalsis.

Arame and hijiki These are the fine, dried strip variety and the mildest flavoured. The strips require soaking in water before being added to salads and cooked dishes.

Dulse Another of the seaweed genus which is generous in its supply of iron.

Kombu There are numerous varieties of this; laminaria is the edible one. Commonly used as a seasoning or in making stock.

Nori The nori roll would not be the same without it! Sold in wafer-thin sheets, nori can also be warmed under the grill and crumbled over a stir-fry or rice dish. It is rich in taurine.

Wakami Wakami is a valuable immune system booster. A good additive to soups, and noodle and rice dishes.

Caution People with thyroid problems should check with their therapist before eating sea vegetables or kelp products.

SEEDS AND NUTS Seeds from the sesame, sunflower and pumpkin provide B complex and other B vitamins, vitamins A, D and E, unsaturated fats, proteins, calcium, fluorine, iodine, iron, magnesium, phosphorus, potassium and zinc. Sunflower seeds can contain as much as 50 per cent protein; sesame seeds are wonderful providers of calcium. Linseed is the best natural source of omega-3 fatty acids.

As with any grain or seed, rancidity can set in immediately the germ is exposed to the air. There is better value in the unhulled varieties, as they can be stored for longer periods. Hulled seeds should be refrigerated and used within a few weeks of harvesting, to avoid the oxidisation of their fat content that will also result in rancidity.

Seeds can be roasted and used as seasonings and snacks. Watermelon seeds plucked from the ripe fruit should never be discarded: they are an excellent source of vitamin E and essential fats, selenium, zinc and protein. Spread them out in a thin layer on any surface where they can be exposed to the sun, to dry. The juice that sticks to them will provide a sweet, tasty crystalline coating for a naturally sun-roasted, cracking good snack. There is no harm in processing the seeds with the pulp when making a refreshing watermelon juice.

Whereas seeds are the ripened ovules of a plant, nuts are the dry fruits, usually of a tree. They provide nutrients similar to seeds, with the addition of copper. Walnuts and hazelnuts are especially rich in essential fatty acids. Nuts require similar storage conditions.

Food substances in seeds and nuts are highly concentrated. Eat them in small quantities as over-eating can place a larger than desired demand on the digestive system. It is essential to chew them thoroughly as small portions can become held over in the small folds of the intestine, leading to decay and auto-intoxication.

SELENIUM This essential mineral has an important role in preventative medicine as a natural antioxidant that protects against free radicals and preserves tissue elasticity. This has a particular relevance to psoriatics of advancing years, as selenium can delay the oxidisation of polyunsaturated fatty acids which play an important role in changes in hormone production and hormone receptor activity.

Selenium is necessary for the production of prostaglandins (substances which influence blood pressure), works with vitamin E in amino acid metabolism, the production of antibodies, in promoting normal growth and fertility, and in binding with toxic metals.

Selenium content in natural sources is affected adversely by sulphur; both fertilisers and acid rain deplete its normal soil levels. Selenium in food is reduced by up to 75 per cent through refining, cooking, processing and heating.

SILICON-CONTAINING FOODS Grapefruit is amongst the 'silicon' foods which are alkali-forming. Silicon in the diet is essential for healthy skin, nails and hair. Oats are high in silicon. (See also *Table 7* in *Appendix 1*.)

SOY PRODUCTS Enter the great soy debate. Recent discoveries have raised serious questions about the benefits or otherwise of soy products. For several decades the soybean, which shares the same family heritage as the largely indigestible peanut, seemed to be the answer to the vegetarian's need to replace meat protein with a non-animal source of protein. Not only was a generation of babies fed on soy compounds, but a plethora of soybean-based foods found a large and enthusiastic market amongst affluent Westerners. Soy milk has replaced cow's milk in millions of households.

The questions arose with the news that soy products can be responsible for severe health derangements, including the blocking of the uptake of calcium, copper, magnesium, iron and zinc in the intestinal tract.[6]

Anyone with a hypothyroid condition should also be aware that the soybean can suppress thyroid function, due to the goitrogens present in the bean.

Soybeans are also one of the crops which feature largely in the debate over genetic modification of foods. Most soybeans derived from major commercial producers are not in their natural genetic state. In addition to their sale in fresh and dried forms, the mutants are used in a very long list of food products that includes baked goods, cooking oils, butter substitutes, confectionary, medicines, vitamins, ice creams, sauces, stocks, shortenings, infant formulas, cheeses and pasta. If you can deal with this factor, soybeans in their various forms—flour, grits, tofu and cultured products—can provide a rich source of alternatives to meat and milk. Soy provides the co-enzyme Q_{10}, phytoestrogens, especially inositol hexaphosphate, an invaluable isoflavone (see page 165), and the protease inhibitor Bowman-Birk inhibitor (BBI).[7]

The Japanese consume soy products as a part of a comprehensive diet that does not include dairy products. Complications with soy in the Western diet can arise when they are bound in combination with dairy and other saturated fats. For the psoriatic, the implication is that some unfermented soy products can be indigestible, especially for those with sensitive digestive systems. The exceptions are to be found in the fermented soy products miso and tamari, or shoyu.

According to some researchers (see *Electrical Nutrition*, pages 190–191), tofu is a non-food. Others argue that, contrary to popular belief, tofu contains no protein, and tofu and bean curd are *deficient* in calcium, magnesium, iron and zinc, in contradiction of analysis by Nutrition Search Inc.[8]

Meanwhile, here are some brief descriptions of the various soy foods.

Miso A cultured soybean product, sold in paste form. High in salt, it is a worthwhile substitute for stock cubes in soups, sauces and gravies.

Soy drinks As an alternative to dairy milk, soy milk is cholesterol-free but requires calcium fortification to lay claim to being calcium-enriched. Used in the manufacture of tofu and some yoghurts.

Soy flour Ground, roasted soybeans. Gluten-free.

Soy sauce, shoyu and tamari Soy sauce is prepared from fermented soybeans and a roasted grain. In addition to its ubiquitous presence on the Chinese restaurant table, soy sauce is used to flavour and season sauces and soups. Shoyu has a slightly mellower flavour, and is prepared from fermented and aged soybeans, and roasted and crushed grain (usually wheat). Tamari is the Japanese variety, made from fermented soybeans and rice. It is usually wheat-free, and has a stronger flavour than shoyu.

Tofu Curdled soy liquid is made into a soft, crumbly cheese-like block. Quite bland in its natural flavour, it responds well to marinating or dipping in shoyu and tamari. It is used in soups, stir-fries and desserts.

Tempeh Another fermented product, tempeh is firmer than tofu and can be used in the same ways. It is a rich source of vitamin B_{12}.

SPROUTS Living food, a fabulous source of enzymes, and literally vibrating with energy. These can be grown from scratch on the tiniest kitchen's window-sill, although there is hardly a fruit and vegetable seller these days who does not offer at least one type of sprouts. Alfalfa sprouts are a good alkaline-forming food.

WATER Skin healers—everybody—should drink six to eight large glasses of fresh, pure water every day. We should be able to do this with confidence, knowing that the water with which we are supplied is fresh and pure. Where this is not the case, consideration should be given to the benefits of spring or distilled water supplies for drinking. Very many varieties of water filtering systems are also available, some of which will remove many, most or all of the impurities present in most municipal water supplies, while some others are a waste of money. Filtering is highly recommended, if only to remove fluoride and chlorine, neither of which was ever intended for human ingestion; indeed, chlorinated water eradicates much of the beneficial bacteria in our bodies. All of these toxins are cumulative.

Taking water a minimum of ten to fifteen minutes prior to a meal is good practice, because it flushes out the stomach and prepares it for fresh inhabitants, and assists with the chemistry of digestion. The colon extracts water from solids and therefore requires water to assist with the process of elimination.

Grapefruit and grape seed extract are used by travellers to treat suspect drinking and cooking water supplies. Liquid chlorophyll can also be added to drinking water from the tap when it is overly chlorinated and repellent for this reason. This is not the only reason to add chlorophyll to drinking water, however. It is a very beneficial substance, as described above.

Dehydration is a very real issue in society at large. It is a common fallacy to assume that because one drinks copious quantities of liquid in the form of tea, coffee or soft drinks each day, sufficient water is being obtained. Because caffeine is present in the majority of these drinks, kidney function is stimulated, with the flushing out of water from the body being one of the results. Water retention is a further factor to be considered. Salt works to retain water in the body. Observe also the preconditions of temperature required for proper digestion and enzyme activity. Taking ice-cold drinks, including water, is not good practice; optimum drinking temperature is 50–68°F (10–20°C).

Mineral waters can provide useful quantities of essential minerals, but aerated and carbonated versions have been shown to be detrimental to the psoriatic condition.

Clay taken internally with uncontaminated (read non-chlorinated) water will provide its wonderful antibacterial, energising, cleansing and re-mineralising properties. It is effective against intestinal parasites, rejuvenates cells and helps restore digestive system balance, extracts toxins, and stimulates and fortifies the immune system. Its high mineral content will effectively deal with mineral deficiencies. Follow the directions for preparations in terms of strength, and duration of the therapy. It is recommended that people with severe or chronic constipation, high blood pressure and hiatus hernia fix those problems before using clay internally.

Other things to be considered

Cooking methods
The way food is prepared can mean the difference between gaining maximum benefit from it, or largely destroying the nutritive value present in the raw food. Generally, 'wet' cooking (steaming) is preferable to 'dry' cooking (e.g. baking). Never boil vegetables; try poaching or braising; shallow-frying instead of deep-frying; grilling instead of frying at all. Minimise cooking time if baking or casseroling at minimum temperature.

Good dietary habits
Avoid drinking anything with or immediately after a meal. The fluid will dilute digestive juices, which is likely to lead to heartburn and stomach discomfort. Soup is an exception to this rule.

Eat raw foods before cooked foods for a healthier immune system. The reasoning behind this is as follows. After cooked food is eaten, white blood cells increase in the intestines. As the immune system automatically stimulates the production of white blood cells to eliminate hostile invaders, this is a certain indicator of the precursors of disease. The creation of white blood cells following the ingestion of cooked food is thus an indication of strain being placed on the immune system. Eating raw food does not cause this production of white blood cells. In fact it has been found that eating raw food before a cooked meal prevents the appearance of white blood cells that would normally occur if only the cooked food was taken. The classic 'salad as a starter' is actually very sound immune system practice. Raw vegetables should be thoroughly chewed, and it is mere common sense that grains and seeds should be treated the same way.

Food temperature is important, too—warm food helps with the process of digestion. The digestive process is also stimulated by oily food, but the choice of oil is important. Seed oils and olive oil have already been discussed; in addition to benefiting digestion, they are good for the complexion.

Food is meant to be taken sitting down. Standing up to eat is antithetical to the relaxed state that should grace a healthy meal. It also encourages a hurried meal, whereas careful, contemplative chewing better facilitates the digestive process. It's also possible to eat too slowly, which impairs digestion because of the irregular enzyme activity. Sleeping straight after a meal, or indulging in vigorous exercise, does not promote proper assimilation.

Stimulating condiments

Spicy condiments—chilli, paprika and mustard—stimulate an increase in gastric juice secretions and can cause irritation to the gut lining or make an existing irritation worse. Ordinarily, the stomach secretes a mucus that protects the lining from irritants. On the good side, chillies are beneficial anticoagulants, and are antioxidants because of their beta-carotene and vitamin C content. The heat of a chilli is attributed to its capsaicin content, which is especially concentrated in the seeds and white rib of the flesh. This compound reduces low-density lipoprotein (LDL) cholesterol, a nasty implicated in heart disease. Endorphins are also released by the brain in response to the burning sensation.

Sensitive digestive systems can be irritated by stimulating condiments such as cayenne pepper, chilli, cinnamon, horseradish, mustard, paprika and pepper (black, white, green and pink).

Cooking utensils

Stainless steel and cast iron cookware are best for use on the stove-top, earthenware for use in the oven, but Pyrex and glass are okay, too. Dispense with aluminium and non-stick varieties, and enamel products that become chipped. Stir and mix with wooden implements.

There is a very good reason for referring to microwave cooking as 'nuking'. Microwaving radically rearranges a food's molecular structure.

Vitamin and mineral supplements

There are two diametrically opposed schools of thought when it comes to the need for or efficacy of vitamin and mineral supplements. When the ordinary dietary intake is devoid of fresh raw fruits and vegetables, or metabolic, endocrinal and gastrointestinal upsets or deficiencies underpin a vitamin or mineral deficiency, there is plain need for supplementation. To a certain extent, of course, the proliferation of vitamin and mineral labels reflects the effectiveness of promotion and the development of a haphazardly pill-popping market that slavishly feeds corporate conglomerates. Worse than this, amidst the hype there is the fact that supplemental intake is harmful to some people.

Some vitamin and mineral claims are indeed a pure scam. According to the Australian Consumers Association (a consumer 'watchdog'), PABA (para-amino-benzoic acid) is such a substance. Some manufacturers claim that PABA is a constituent of the vitamin B group, others that it stimulates intestinal bacteria, breaks down protein, restores greying hair, and is a sun block. The Australian Consumers Association refutes this and warns that manufacturers are fully aware not only of the uselessness of the product, but that it can worsen bacterial infections. As an additive to sun blocks in the past, it acted as a phototoxic agent and its use was discontinued. Furthermore, contrary to having any value in this form, it also failed to filter out the sun's rays which cause skin cancer.[9]

While billions of dollars are spent every year on vitamin and mineral supplements, artificial supplementation can in no way compare with the naturally-derived forms of the nutrients. Vitamins and minerals obtained from foods are bound to natural food complexes (carbohydrates, lipids and proteins). In contrast, many vitamin and mineral supplements are not even produced from natural sources—synthetic supplements are exactly that, synthetic. For example, synthetic vitamin D (ergocalciferol) is produced by irradiating the ergosterol in yeast with ultraviolet light. Natural vitamin D (cholecalciferol) is actually a steroid. It is converted by the kidneys into calcitriol, which together with the parathyroid hormone maintains blood levels of calcium and phosphate. The balance of these nutrients in the body is very sensitive, and generally supplementation of vitamin D would not be recommended. When vitamin D is made in the skin, the body has the means of maintaining safe blood levels; when too much is taken orally, a chemical which should be produced via normal metabolism in the intestine and liver reaches toxic levels in the blood.

A potentially dangerous practice in food production is fortification with vitamins and minerals. This raises the question of another very important reason for clear direction in the use of supplements, namely absorption and the body's way of using vitamins and minerals. The ingestion of synthetic vitamin D-fortified milk can increase the discharge of magnesium from the body. Amongst its many essential roles, magnesium is necessary for the production of calcium and vitamin C.

Regardless of how many or what type of supplements we take, if our body does not have the appropriate level or type of enzyme present for dealing with it, the intake will be worthless. Enzymes are essential for the assimilation of these nutrients—the nutrients simply are not activated until they encounter enzymes, whether they be taken in fresh food or supplemental form. Hence the need arises in some people who are suffering from a chronic degenerative condition to also use dietary enzyme supplements.

In a further aspect of food combining, some essential amino acids when taken in supplemental form should not be consumed with milk or other high-protein foods, as they will compete for the same receptor points.

The best advice will be based on individual assessment by a qualified practitioner.

Deconditioning

Instead of being conditioned to regard 'health food'—read real food—as strange,[10] we could be conditioned to prefer it; or to opt for it because we want to do ourselves a favour. We are conditioned by education, the media and our upbringing, and even by those who are both near and distant to us, to accept certain criteria as being 'normal'. Anything that doesn't conform is 'strange' or 'weird', usually inferior. This concept is applied across the spectrum of human existence, whether it be to food preferences, clothing styles, personality, race, religion and philosophy, even the job one has or doesn't have. Yet, with the input of accurate conditioning a disclaimer is easily transformed into a proclaimer, or a calm humanitarian into a programmed assassin.

In properly treating psoriasis, to achieve de-conditioning—detoxifying, eliminating—could require re-conditioning our mindset, re-examining attitudes, becoming accepting of an open approach to new ideas and concepts. Presumption and supposition have no place to settle in deconditioned thinking; there is room for everybody and everything. Neither is there fear or anxiety, for love can support all and faith can guide destiny.

At some time or another we have to grapple with taste conditioning before new foods or medicines are palatable. Time works wonders. So does understanding. For example, many readers will now have a better understanding of psoriasis—indeed, of illness—than before they opened this book. This has overcome conditioning that 'very little is known about psoriasis …' New conditioning has taken its place, not the least from the declaration '… many readers will now have a better understanding …' This is similar to an advertising ploy—or conditioning—which implants a suggestion, be it positive or otherwise.

It seems there is little escape from conditioning, other than to maintain an awareness of it and be alert to its many negative repercussions. The overriding principles are to remain open to new ideas, to spend time and thought in their evaluation, and to exercise free will in determining their efficacy or appropriateness, and therefore level of acceptance.

Regaining balance

Healing a leaky gut

Decontamination and remedial action are at the core of arresting this decline of the digestive system.

Fresh vegetables and fruits are the most important dietary therapy in addressing the unusually permeable intestines prevalent amongst psoriatics.

Oil, particularly virgin olive oil is beneficial. Herbal teas, notably chamomile and mullein, can also be beneficial. So too can a glass of water with a pinch of slippery elm powder stirred in, and taken before eating breakfast.

To be avoided, as they are detrimental to the condition, are fried foods, red meat, pork and ham, excess carbohydrate, and more than one type of starch in any one meal, excess fat, sugar combined with carbohydrate, and spicy condiments.

Acids and alkalis

An acid/alkaline balance of the blood is fundamental to good health, whether or not we suffer from psoriasis. A psoriatic will probably have an acidic blood balance.

In the 1930s, Dr Howard Hay deduced that people with an acidic blood balance were more likely to suffer ill health. His research into health and nutrition enabled the formulation of dietary rules that centred on proper food combinations.[11]

Acid-forming and alkaline-forming foods

Our intake of mineral salts—calcium, magnesium, potassium and sodium—affects our blood acid/alkaline balance. Fresh vegetables provide rich sources of these mineral salts. Raw fruits are highly alkaline. (See also *Table 8* in *Appendix 1*.)

Foods with a high content of chlorine, phosphorus, sulphur and nitrogen weigh on the acid-forming side. Animal products are such foods; so again, we find a sound reason for limiting, or eliminating altogether, land animal protein and foods produced with or containing animal products. However, it should be noted that all minerals to some degree are necessary in the body system. For example, chlorine foods are important in the psoriatic's diet. The saltiness of tears and perspiration is chlorine, and it is called for to repair cracked nails and dull skin. Chlorine promotes the absorption of new blood material and the transfer of waste products from tissues to the blood. Without chlorine in the system, impurities and germs would remain in the body.

Differentiation needs to be made between the mineral as a nutrient (such as provided in a natural food source) and the chemical as an artificially produced substance that finds its way into the body system. For example, to drink chlorinated tap water is to invite oxidisation and the destruction of vitamins C and E. In a similar sense, whilst copper is a necessary trace element in the balanced body, it can be in excess as the result of its entry via artificial means. Excessive plasma copper levels are often found in psoriatics. This can be the result of heavy metal poisoning, but more important perhaps is its possible role in irritation of the gastrointestinal tract.

Food combining

If the food we buy and eat is nutritionally ill-affected by production and processing methods, it is vital that all surviving nutritive value is allowed to endure the digestive process.

Diligent food combining can be really hard core, most likely committed to the too-hard basket by most people, conditioned as we are to preferred tastes, favourite dishes and blended flavours. Even when deciding to knuckle down and observe some basic rules, it is so very easy to allow these rules to lapse. Nevertheless we should strive to know and understand the basic principles of food combining and refuse to accept as normal that indigestion is the result of meal-taking.

It is of further interest to note that exercise makes the blood more acidic, while deep breathing makes the blood more alkaline. Exercise is essential for good health. It depends on what we are hoping to achieve, however. A pleasant walk in a calm space—a forest, gardens, a beach—is less stressful than a jog on asphalt. A couple of hours in the garden can be more therapeutic and a sounder work out, than two hours of straining and stressing in the gym. (See also *Tables 9* and *10* in *Appendix 1*.)

Yeast infection

When gut bacteria are destroyed by antibiotics, the body will probably experience an overgrowth of a yeast-like organism. This unwanted guest can be helped along by a diet high in sugar, including fructose from fruit. Antifungal agents such as grape seed or grapefruit extract can be highly effective.

Yeast is present in bakery goods, vinegar and foods that contain vinegar (e.g. mayonnaise and many sauces), alcoholic and fermented beverages, and products which contain yeast-derived vitamins of the B complex. The leaves of black tea are yeast-fermented. Torula yeast is a fungus; and yeast is also present in the classic fungus, the mushroom. It is also present in olives, malted products (including canned citrus and fruit juices, not to mention breakfast cereals) and tomato sauce.

In addition to sugar and refined flour, the yeast bacteria is promoted by alcohol, blue cheese, bread, coffee, chocolate, honey, maple syrup, mushrooms, MSG, smoked foods, tea and vinegar.

Yoghurt, olive oil and garlic are essential in the battle against yeast infection. In addition, in a series of studies of psoriatic patients treated with oral nystatin for yeast infection such as *Candida albicans*, remarkable remission was achieved.[12] A nutritionist will conduct the necessary tests and identify the extent, if any, of 'your' infection.

Antioxidants

Loftiest amongst the nutrient antioxidants, in the vitamin regime at least, is vitamin C. It, along with A, E, zinc, selenium, iron, manganese and copper are vital forces against oxidising chemicals, or free radicals. Vitamin A promotes health in the digestive and respiratory tracts. As a water-soluble vitamin, C provides protection from the inside of the cell; the fat-soluble vitamin E and beta-carotene provide protection to the cell's fatty membrane.

Research is constantly uncovering new antioxidants, substances which are categorised as non-nutrient antioxidants, namely bioflavenoids, carotenoids, phytochemicals and polyphenols. These are all essential in warding off infection and are effective in slowing down the ageing process. The immune system of a toxic psoriatic body is sure to be imbalanced in favour of scavenging free radicals, and therefore in urgent need of harmonising antioxidant action.

Essential food sources of antioxidants include soybeans, oatmeal products, berry fruits, the spices turmeric, allspice and cloves, the herbs horseradish, oregano, parsley, rosemary, sage and thyme, and fresh, vital fruits and vegetables.

Cysteine, an amino acid with a direct relationship with taurine, is another powerful antioxidant. Together with glutathione, cysteine helps with the production of glutathione peroxidase, one of the body's main antioxidising enzymes. Glutathione peroxidase is in turn dependent on selenium, which helps to detoxify the body and to promote the immune system. Psoriatics generally exhibit very low levels of glutathione peroxidase. Vitamin E restores this essential enzyme to optimal levels, and pantothenic acid (vitamin B_5) increases its levels.

Natural antibody production is dependent upon the presence of vitamin B_6. It is also essential for T cell production. Vitamin B_{12} and folic acid are also essential to the proper functioning of T cells. Similarly zinc has an essential role in the production of immune cells. Some psoriatics have been found to be deficient in zinc, and have demonstrated success in gaining remission when introducing zinc supplements to their vitamin and mineral intake.

Factors and substances which suppress the immune system include vigorous exercise, corticosteroids, stress, depression and grief.

Factors and substances which enhance the immune system include calming, non-stressful exercise, relaxation, meditation and adequate intake of appropriate vitamins and minerals (A, B_1, B_2, B_6, B_{12}, folic acid, C, E, iron, zinc, magnesium, selenium).

Melatonin is one of the most efficient agents against free radicals. In its homeopathic form it can be beneficial as an antioxidant, in helping to provide stamina and endurance, and to relieve stress, nervous tension, anxiety, and insomnia.

Importantly, the essential and non-essential antioxidants work most effectively when they are present together in a balanced form, rather than as separate entities. In addition, the amino acids, peptides and proteins that are made available through the digestion of any food containing protein, have a synergistic relationship with antioxidants.

Other non-essential antioxidants are carotenoids, phytochemicals, phytoestrogens and polyphenols.

- *Carotenoids* are many and varied, and include beta-carotene, glutathione, quercetin, lutein and lycopene.
- *Phytochemicals* (also known as *isoflavones*) are provided in many fresh fruits and vegetables. In their various compound forms, these substances have been recognised as being highly effective in detoxification processes, and (as antioxidants) in intercepting and

dealing summarily with toxins and carcinogens.

Tomatoes possess approximately 10,000 phytochemicals. However, commercially-grown tomatoes present the raw food aficionado with a major dilemma, in so far as the inordinate number of pests and diseases working against tomato cropping result in a veritable deluge of pesticides, herbicides and fertilisers. In addition to their toxic cloak, for ages now tomatoes have been genetically modified to forestall their natural habit of ripening (before hitting the shelf).

Apart from tomatoes, lecithin, lignans (such as are found in linseed oil and milk thistle), omega-3 fatty acids and saponins (such as are found in sarsaparilla) provide these highly beneficial substances. They are also found in numerous other sources, including coumarins and flavenoids (present in vegetables and fruits, and bee pollen), and allium compounds (found in onions and garlic). Another class of phytochemical, phenolic acids, is found in ginger, onions, oats, red wine, grapes and various other fruits (especially citrus) and vegetables. Ginger root (of the same botanical family as sage, rosemary, oregano and thyme—the *Labiatae*) is extremely rich in phenolic compounds.

- *Phytoestrogens* are present in large amounts in soybeans and their related products. These compounds have been found in high levels in the blood of women with lower levels of strong oestrogen in their bodies.
- *Polyphenols* are provided in some fruits and vegetables, nuts, wine, coffee and tea. In particular, green tea is a source of the polyphenols that work with vitamins C and E to protect the skin from ultraviolet light, to burn body fat and promote cholesterol balance, and provide antioxidant defence against, and foraging of, free radicals.

Note that the antioxidants listed as additives on product packaging are not of the same class as these described above. (See also *Table 11* in *Appendix 1*.)

Additional factors

Real people don't need hamburger

How much protein does the average human body require daily? If each individual is unique, with organs of different shapes and sizes, different metabolic rates, and different needs for vitamins and minerals, there can be no straightforward answer to this question. The standard answers of conventional or orthodox dietetic advice are informed by thinking which has its foundation in models devised by the US Department of Agriculture in the late 1950s, in response to the need to support marketing initiatives by the three main food producers, the cattle, dairy and grain industries.[13]

What is good protein? The availability of 25 amino acids in the different forms of food protein is fundamental to body growth and repair; they are instrumental in the production of antibodies, enzymes, hormones and neurotransmitters. The balance of these amino acids determines the quality of the protein, and therefore the ability of the machine, the body, to function.

From our youngest days we have it drummed into our beliefs and attitudes that the best way to obtain protein is from animal sources. These sources also provide too much unwanted saturated fat—anathema to the healing psoriatic. Offal should be avoided at all costs, because it contains the essential fatty acid arachidonic acid, which irritates psoriasis because it is converted to pro-inflammatory prostaglandins. Healthful supplies of protein are available from non-animal food sources, which simultaneously provide other constituent nutritive factors beneficial to the process of skin repair and generally sound bodily constitution.

Excess meat produces calcium deficiency. Imbalance occurs in the body in the presence of inadequate levels of calcium. The production of ammonia, sluggishness, general over-acidity and the onset of intestinal putrefaction can be the result of excess animal protein in the diet. Every day, people die with chunks of undigested meat lodged in their intestines.

The ready availability of fast foods—hamburgers, fried chicken, pizzas, combined with carbonated, sugar-loaded or excitotoxin-riddled beverages—and their consumption at all levels of society does not augur well for a healthy society, let alone encourage sensible dietary practice for the healing psoriatic. Who knows, could the use of growth hormones to produce fatter (and hence more profitable) creatures for slaughter to feed the fast-food faddists one day see hamburger-chomping he-men sprouting breasts? Impotence, infertility and mortally deficient immune systems might be hailed as the hallmarks of non-discerning meat-eaters.

Above all, forsake the fast-food takeaway in the name of health, and help realise benefits far and beyond remission.

Who's tampering with our food?

To our shame and our detriment, our soils have been utterly depleted by fertilisers and herbicides, irrigation and erosion. Some soils have been knowingly sterilised—the large tracts of land in Vietnam on which the defoliants Agent Orange (and Agents White, Pink, Blue, Green and Purple) were bombed during the war. Soil sterilants and picloram, which has a long-term residual effect in the soil, were key ingredients in these defoliants.[14] In the 1940s, people who worked in plants manufacturing dioxin (2,4,5-T), aka Agent Orange et al., contracted chloracne as a result of industrial accidents.[15]

Those who were responsible for manufacturing these agents have bought up seed stocks. By creating hybrids, and genetically modifying plants to produce strains that must be sprayed by their own herbicides, these same entities have created an emasculating loop to the detriment of all but themselves. The raw food materials are then processed beyond recognition.

Granted that a calculated degree of preservation of foods for mass consumption is necessary to get them to the marketplace in sufficient quantities to fulfil the needs for fast-moving consumer goods (FMCG)—but why do things like aspartame have to be introduced? If synthetic sweeteners have to replace sugar, why does sugar have to be replaced? That's right, it's fattening. And it has been implicated in some diseases. Why is there so much tampering with our sustenance; why is there so much devotion to perfecting substances that are widely known to be harmful?

Are we too clever for our own good?

Is our food capable of keeping up with us?

Alternatives

It is one thing to learn of foods and substances that are detrimental to the process of healing psoriasis and achieving a quality of life without the disease constantly dragging us down. It is quite another to know how to address these changes without having to lapse into a bland diet that can make dining a singularly uninteresting experience. Sitting down to a meal should be a pleasurable experience one looks forward to, especially if one is also involved in the preparation of the meal. A very important part of the digestive and assimilation processes is this sense of enjoyment, and appreciation of the benefits of the food that is being taken. Thinking positively about the foods as we chew and enjoy them is a very necessary process. We might even go so far as to expect that this active application of our mental attitude could help promote the benefits.

It might be useful to learn of some alternatives to the foods, beverages and condiments that are best avoided. In many cases, it may be a matter of developing new tastes. This can require perseverance and dedication, depending upon the degree of change it will mean to the regular diet. Many of the alternative foods and substances listed here can represent an acquired taste. Given the very real benefits of pursuing this course, however, it can be worthwhile persevering to develop that acquired taste.

ALCOHOL The ethanol in alcohol increases the absorption of toxins in the gastrointestinal tract and impairs liver function. Being a vasodilator, alcohol will widen blood vessels and increase the blood flow to the skin. Alcohol also stimulates the production of uric acid.

On the other hand, ethanol increases levels of high-density lipoprotein (HDL) cholesterol, the good-guy cholesterol that is a protector against heart disease. Also, wine contains polyphenols (flavenoids) that destroy bacteria (brandy was used to kill typhoid and cholera germs in the nineteenth century). Generally, aged red wine is more beneficial than young white wine, because it has undergone a longer fermentation process, during which the antibacterial properties have been fully developed; therefore the older the vintage, the more powerful its antioxidant qualities. While its age will probably add to the wine's cost, a general rule of thumb anyway is that the cheaper the wine, the more it has been chemically tampered with. 'Drier' wines contain more tannin, also an indication of greater benefits.

There are some fabulous wines produced from organically grown grapes, but most still contain preservatives, while there are preservative-free non-organic wines.

Unless you feel that non-alcoholic drinks are a substitute for alcohol, there is no alternative except to find a low-alcohol alcoholic drink. 'Light' beer is still going to introduce carbonation and other irritants; wine is wine and spirits are spirits. Moderation still seems to be the only real alternative, although complete abstention should be at least attempted during the initial and determined phases of a general and complete clean-out (and unquestionably during pregnancy).

ANIMAL PROTEINS (MEAT) Vegetarians obtain sufficient protein for amino acid conversion from a balanced diet comprising rice, legumes, pulses, beans, cereal grains, nuts, seeds, fermented cultures and vegetables. Some cultured dairy products (yoghurt, cottage cheese, ricotta cheese) can supplement protein requirements in those who are not indisposed to them. Find a metabolic type and stick to it, as they say. Consult a naturopath or nutritionist or someone who is capable of providing equally sound dietetic advice and who practises wholistically.

To the carnivore nothing replaces the need to chew flesh or quells the craving for charred meat and blood. Some metabolic types quite naturally require protein from animal sources. It is expected that certified organic meat is better quality and safer to eat than non-organic meat. Moderation, and the application of sound dietary rules and practices, can be the key to achieving a balanced state if animal proteins are to continue to be a part of your diet.

Fish from the deep sea is preferable to coastal catches because of their oil content and the lesser likelihood of contamination by pollutants resulting from agricultural, sewerage and urban effluents.

Seek out sources of organic, free-range chicken if poultry takes your fancy, and apply the same principles to the consumption of eggs. In addition to deriving sustenance from comparatively untainted meat, you will be contributing to more humane practices.

BLACK TEA There are any number of caffeine-free herbal teas on the market these days.

In addition to its alkaloidal caffeine content, ordinary tea contains theophylline, a nervous system irritant that is five times more potent than the caffeine. The astringent tannins in tea prejudice digestive enzyme secretion, contribute to constipation and hinder iron absorption. Coffee, tea and cocoa all contain the drug theobromine.

There are actually three tea categories—black, green and oolong. Black tea is fermented; green is unfermented; oolong is semi-fermented. Green tea also contains caffeine, but a lesser amount. Both green and black tea are antioxidants, although green tea's antioxidant power is six times greater than black tea's. Note, however, that the addition of milk to either type negates its antioxidant properties. Pregnant women should not consume more than five cups of green tea per day.

BREAD (YEASTED) The benefits of sourdough breads were discussed on page 142.

BUTTER, MARGARINE Replace with vegetable, seed and nut oil-based spreads, and avocado.

COFFEE Cereal coffees, although usually an unsatisfactory alternative for anyone who really enjoys fresh, full-flavoured coffee, are readily available.

Dandelion coffee is 'good medicine' as it increases liver activity and that of the pancreas and spleen, and assists with the digestion of fats. In fact, the whole plant has powerful antioxidant qualities, as it possesses high levels of vitamins A and C. The dandelion root is dried and ground, and in its granulated form is perfect for the espresso, percolator, etc. A rich and satisfying drink can be made which may be combined with milk or cream and sugar, or however you like your poison.

While they might not be practical for the majority of coffee drinkers, the methods for preparing true Arabian coffee and Turkish coffee weaken the caffeine content. In the authentic way, the beans are freshly roasted and ground as required, the brew is rapidly boiled and served with the grounds.

CONDIMENTS (SAUCES) Replace tomato sauce, black sauce, barbecue sauce and other such pre-prepared mixtures with tamari (also known as shoyu), soy sauce (check the ingredients and avoid brands which contain caramel and MSG, usually listed as additive 621) and organic seasonings in powdered and bouillon forms.

COW'S MILK Drink water. Cow's milk is best left to baby cows.[16]
Milk contains at least 20 proteins, and the psoriatic, let alone a large portion of humanity, has considerable difficulty with their digestion. I am not referring to milk sugar, which is another and separate matter for allergenics altogether.

Goat's milk, and milks made from oats and almonds, can be very worthwhile substitutes.

FATTY AND OILY FOODS Sluggish liver and gall bladder action will result from a preponderance of fatty and oily foods. Stay away from the take-away.

IODISED TABLE SALT Salt is necessary for homeostasis. The chlorine in common table salt (sodium chloride) can present a problem for the skin. Chlorine is separated in the body from sodium and experiences little assimilation through metabolism. Leftover chlorine is stored in the connective tissues, and has a particular affinity for the cells directly beneath the skin surface.

Suitable alternatives are evaporated sea salt, rock salt, vegetable salt and kelp powder or granules.

SWEETS, DESSERTS It is more a question of when to have these than of finding alternatives. The practice of concluding a meal with a sweet cold dessert followed by hot coffee is tantamount to making a firm and conscious decision to have a problem with your digestion. Given a rudimentary understanding of the digestive processes, suddenly swamping the combination of starch, protein and sugars already in the stomach with hot, cold, and more hot substances seems a rather strange thing to do.

But they're hard to give up, aren't they? Carob cannot replace chocolate for the so-called chocoholic; cheesecake is cheesecake is cheesecake; mother *would* forgive if we forsook the tiramisu or apple pie. You deal with it.

Food as energy

All matter is energy. This is recognised by the alternative healing modalities which endeavour to treat the person wholistically. The vibrationary rate, discernible and measurable in the aura, or energy body, will be much different in a seriously diseased person to that of a person in the peak of health. The higher vibratory rate is visible in 'glowing good health'. Determined action to achieve a positive healing state can directly influence the vibration.

Personal, individual energy is hard-wired to the universal life-force or energy. Homeopathy and the subtle healing arts understand this and work with it (see pages 181–183).

Raw fresh food radiates greater levels of vibration than cooked food, while food that has been irradiated imbues an altogether different manifestation of this radiation; it is definitely not on the 'positive' side.

8 Within and without

All diseases of the body proceed from the mind or soul.

Plato

The mind's role in dis-ease

As psoriatics we can rigorously pursue the perfect healthy diet, but if we harbour inappropriate mental or attitudinal conditioning we might just as well smear our bodies with tar and eat supermarket food exclusively. A healthy perspective on life is essential. The mind must be nourished equally with the body in the pursuit of balance, for thought, emotion and memory automatically engender chemical and electrical activity which results in powerful coded information coursing throughout the whole body system.

A deterioration in health can be easily brought about by negative emotions and thought patterns, with stress, resentment, nervousness and hatred being major culprits. Fear and tension (stress) produce automatic physiological reactions—extra adrenalin is produced by the adrenal gland, heartbeat and respiration accelerate, blood pressure rises, and the liver receives an extra dose of glucose. Fear, embarrassment and pleasure can change our skin temperature, cause sebaceous glands to secrete more heavily, and stimulate blood vessels to send a sudden rush of supplies to the body's surface.

Attitude

Let's put everything we know about the body behind us; forget about metabolic, endocrinal, autoimmune and genetic factors in our wonderful state of dis-ease. After all, their importance—and indeed their reality—is irrelevant because we have *decided* to have this problem. It could not exist without our conscious or sub-conscious decision to allow it; everything else we do is intended to support or flow on from this decision. So imagine if we decided to *not* have it?

Surely, if we decided to have this disease psoriasis, ultimately we could determine how well or unwell we were going to be? The genuinely religious or spiritual individual can get by on pure faith; yet how many of us place our faith in science, technology or, worse still, leadership, while we give scant consideration to signing over our personal power to the unseen? Is our attention meant to be swept up in sensory perception? We are thinking, feeling, spiritual entities nourished and affected by our thoughts, the imposition of others' attitudes and viewpoints, disaffected by authority, and soothed and manipulated by faiths, concepts and beliefs. We are the superior animal amongst a myriad of life forms, yet we can be conditioned and manipulated to within a breath's distance from the robotic.

It is easy to be conditioned—it can start in the womb, where a food allergy can be introduced. Our sexual preferences can be developed in the womb too, and not as a product of our home life, according to the authors of a book called *BrainSex*.[1] From the moment we are born, the expectation is on us to conform with certain standards and conditions. Viewed historically, education has been used for mind control at its worst and to promote competition.

Amidst educated thought emerge social engineering and eugenics. We accept addiction as a fact of life, whether it be to drugs, megalomania or even a religion. In a quest for identity, succour, we can lose the same personal power we give away as when accepting a bone-pointing medico's declaration that our disease is terminal or incurable. For all of its good, mainstream religion has inculcated a belief in the necessity for guilt, and given excuses for genocide and racism. Will steadfast political correctness really address these issues?

There is no shortage of information available about proper nutrition and the critical roles of diet and lifestyle in health and in disease, but more and more we remain content in the belief that some or other drug or medication is being developed—if not already available—to 'cure' this illness. So we feed on the garbage heap and assign our lives to the control of other people and lifeless concepts. Such is the stupidity of our beliefs, which we allow because we have lost sight of the fact that we each possess a truly mighty instrument, the power of thought. It is uniquely our own. We can apply it to get well. Step one is making this affirmative decision and letting go of the rest. It is essential to maintain a firm desire for, and expectation of, being healed.

How thoughts work

The thinking process depends on the brain's state of wakefulness. It rouses the entire brain into activity by the stimulation of the upper portions of the region in the brain stem known as the reticular formation, and particularly the portions which are located in the mesencephalon and upper pons. This system is called the reticular activating system, and it transmits the majority of its signals to the cerebral cortex through the thalamus.

The brain is not exclusively an electrical system; its activity is driven by hormones, the secretions that link communications between the body's cells. Hormones travel from the brain to the endocrine system, and through this to all of the body's organs; it is also known that this is a two-way communication.[2] Hormones or peptides that are manufactured and stored in the brain are identical to those produced in the gut, and in this respect are unique amongst their kind: otherwise each gland (thyroid et al) secretes its own hormones. The brain and intestine can communicate directly with each other, which gives new meaning to the sensation of having a 'gut feeling' about something.

This is also important news for the psoriatic, because it further illustrates how our emotional state influences our immune system, and ultimately our state of health—depression, loneliness and anxiety can have repercussions throughout the body. There is commonsense in adopting a program that embraces some form of positive psychological therapy.

Behavioural patterns—pleasure and reward, pain and punishment—are influenced by the limbic system which governs rage and excitability and love, compliance and even submissiveness.

Some forms of psychoneuroimmunology regard the brain as also being a receiver and amplifier of collective consciousness. Perhaps this could be utilised in the healing process, and in managing well-being to the extent that dis-ease does not have an atmosphere in which to grow.

Lifestyle, relaxation and exercise

Ideally, employment should be more than just a job. As platitudinous as it might have become, it is still true that one should live to work, not work to live. Who really works in a job that feeds their soul?[3] Underlying this is the need to do something for oneself rather than to please or serve others. Better we function on behalf of our own best interests. This is not to practise selfishness, but to recognise our own needs and to fulfil them first in order to be useful (another platitude). After all, our contribution to the employer, home life, the community, the universe can only be worthwhile if our physical, emotional and spiritual selves are healthy.

If each and every one of us has a purpose for being here, it is necessary to know what this is, and through realising it and freely living and pursuing it, really achieve well-being. Only then will we be producing the right chemicals and setting off the correct electrical impulses.

Therefore our lifestyle—private life—should provide opportunities for creativity, rest and reflection. A lifestyle that allows for deep relaxation, such as is achieved through meditation, can also lead to spiritual fulfilment. Similarly, there is greater benefit in regular light exercise than in strenuous gym workouts or body-building. Regular exercise, as slight as it might be, can produce health benefits and prevent disease—in addition to toning muscles, it stimulates digestion, metabolism and nutrient absorption, improves circulation, and aids the elimination of wastes. Light exercise can also elevate one's mood.[4]

Regular yoga exercise and tai chi also work with the subtle energies, developing therapeutic breathing practices, and awakening the meditative state and therefore pathways to self-awareness and inner health. In these, as in any form of exercise, relaxation or activity—prayer, devotion—it is the mind, body and spirit that are being refreshed and nourished.

Meditation and the state of deep relaxation are held as being vital to the support of the immune system and the creation of a space wherein the individual achieves a condition of inner peace, positive feelings, and openness to now. Regular practice will have benefits that cross personal and biological levels, and ultimately lead to an understanding of and experience in the universal intelligence which informs all matter. Similarly, creative visualisation and a straightforward, down to earth, positive determination to overcome, can obtain a chemical adjustment by affecting our immune system. Meditation does not require any belief, faith, visualisation or affirmations, and can lead to a deep awareness and a profound sense of belonging which transcends the material world.

Inner consciousness

We Westerners started looking for this en masse in the 1960s. It seemed like a good idea at the time, although it was particularly higher consciousness that we sought to attain. It must have worked, because human experience has been altered by what we found and the study of consciousness continues to attract interest and funding for research. Then again, maybe we failed miserably, because in late 2000 the World Health Organisation ranked depression as the world's fourth largest cause of disease.[5]

Meanwhile, many non-Western traditional cultures have long known more about higher consciousness than we presently know or will ever know, if we rely only on empirical studies. Traditional insight arises from an innate understanding of the natural laws that govern our existence as expressions of the 'ineffable spark', a concept that Western thought has to grapple with, tied as we are to the need for scientific proof of absolutely everything. Some cultures accept the need to maintain a healthy 'temple' (body) if for no other reason than to observe respect for the mortal body which is held as an expression of the divine 'spark', God, the source of consciousness, indeed the ultimate 'source' itself. This responsibility to maintain good health has filtered through and ultimately must uplift the human experience, and enable a positive and worthwhile contribution to our evolution as a species.

Meanwhile it is not necessary to attain a certain level of perfection or consciousness to do away with psoriasis; it is enough to be open to new thoughts and concepts which could prove extremely worthwhile.

Thinking it away

Hypnotherapy

Do realise that this is not the stage spectacle. Hypnosis is a genuine scientific procedure recognised by most Western medical associations. Applied as a therapeutic tool, hypnosis has nothing to do with titillation, being taken under the control of another person, or wilful submission for that matter. Hypnotherapy is about control, but it is your own control of yourself, your mind and body.

Nobody can be deeply hypnotised against his or her will. The state of hypnosis is a perfectly safe place in which you exist with a complete conscious presence: you remain fully alert and aware of your surroundings, and of the hypnotist's words and instructions. You cannot get locked into a 'trance', for you are not in a trance state; you will not become 'possessed' or 'lost'. Under hypnotherapy, the acceptance (and effect) of suggestions and statements that you make or accept will go much deeper than they would in the non-hypnotic state. It is the power of suggestion that is at work here and its effectiveness is well established.

Hypnotherapy was officially recognised as a medical aid by the British Medical Association in 1955, although its uses were described as early as the 1840s. At this time a French provincial doctor, A. A. Liébault, used hypnotism with positive effect in his daily practice. Two contemporaries of Liébault, Emile Coué and Charles Baudoin, were the earliest exponents of autosuggestion, which took hypnosis to the next and logical step—it obviated the need for the hypnotist and placed the therapeutic role solely in the hands (or mental capacity) of the one receiving the therapy. Hypnosis is also used as an effective alternative to anaesthesia prior to some surgical procedures.

In the 1940s, a clinical study in India described how a patient with an extensive psoriatic body cover was hypnotised. Under hypnosis, the patient was given a series of suggestions, which had a remarkable outcome. One-half of the body was to be 'treated' for the psoriasis, while the other half was to be left 'untreated' as a control. As a result of this, the patient experienced a total remission on the limbs and part of the trunk which received the hypnotic treatment, while the 'untreated' side remained unchanged. A similar experiment was described in the *British Medical Journal* in 1952, wherein a patient with congenital ichthyosis covering much of his body received hypnotic suggestion. The different parts of the body which were to receive treatment were nominated in advance. Those limbs which received 'suggestion' cleared: the scaly, horny layer which characterises this particular skin disease fell away, and the skin cleared to reveal normal, healthy growth. The condition remained unchanged on the limbs that were left 'untreated'.

The hypnotherapist's patient should be a willing and active participant. This is probably true of any form of treatment which does not rely on strong artificial drugs; even then it is more than likely the patent's faith in the scientific, in the 'magic potion', which elevates its effectiveness. As was outlined earlier, the effect of potent steroids and strong topical applications diminishes with time anyway; as surely as the luckless psoriatic's faith in the product must moderate as temporary remission is balanced with the often ghastly side-effects.

While hypnotherapy might reduce the time that successful treatment takes, it does not necessarily mean that the nature of the treatment should be altered. Therefore topical and dietary programs should be pursued and maintained.

In some applications of hypnotherapy, the patient is asked to participate by visualising the patches of psoriasis diminishing in size and 'leaving' the body. Visualisation of this sort is a very powerful tool, with or without the aid of the hypnotic state. It can be practised unaided at any time. All it requires is a calm, quiet space, a state of relaxation, and a clear focus on the matter. Again the underlying principle is a positive mental attitude. This approach can be used when applying natural oils and creams, with the mental image being one of rubbing on an emollient which is actually pleasant to use, on an area of skin which is visualised as becoming healthier, stronger, clearer. This can be far more beneficial and therapeutic than dragging oneself through a routine of applying an expensive, smelly potion to a clearly disturbed area of skin.

Perhaps hypnotherapy could be used to suggest that one develops a liking for certain foods or, maybe more appropriately, to develop a dislike for foods that are deleterious to the psoriatic condition.

The selection of any therapist in whom you are going to place your trust should be based on enquiry into established professional competence and experience. As for medical practitioners and natural therapists, formal associations exist through which reference can be gained to qualified members.

Overall, however, the best form of hypnotherapy would be one which enables you to use it on yourself; so that taking control becomes just that. Ideally, hypnotherapy treatment should automatically lead you to self-hypnosis—this is not something that one should have to rely on another for, because it seems to negate the very purpose for which its help is being sought (taking control).

Visualisation

This is using thought to create a visual impression, an ideal in the mind's eye. Just as thought processes rely on and stimulate brain function, visualisation works in partnership with the body's remarkable self-healing ability to instil a target or goal. Some people swear by the same process for creating success and riches.

Inner listening

If we are in doubt about something, ultimately our inner or higher self is poised to assist. Remember the last time you were puzzled by a problem at work or school and needed 'time to think it over', or decided that you might 'sleep on it'? Some time later, maybe next day, you had the answer, or felt more confident in making a decision. The process of taking time to dwell on the problem was tantamount to consulting your inner self. Some people are very successful at practising like this all the time. Try this: ask yourself to help with the answer to something by concentrating on it in the last moments before going to sleep. On awakening, spend a few quiet moments with the subject again. You should get an immediate and very clear response. This might take a bit of practice, and you will undoubtedly benefit by some further reading on it, but it is a reality and you can usually rely on the 'advice'.

Living as we do in a world which is governed by rationalism, and therefore functions in favour of left-brain activity, we have all but forgotten to use our intuitive (right-brain) selves. (Apparently we are economic rationalists, certainly our laws and mores are logically driven, and we acquire qualifications that are essential for employment, as a result of proving that we are capable of regurgitating someone else's carefully determined facts.) While our intuition might be dormant, it is not dead (it has to be alert in women who possess the remarkable ability to grow and nurture a child). However, by not listening to (using) our natural intuition, another of our connections with the universal life force and mind, we are inviting emotional and mental imbalance.

Creative expression

Creative thought power can be diminished by worry, fear, despair and envy; it can be nurtured and enhanced by expressing, flexing and exercising intuition and free expression in any form that takes our fancy. Suppression of the freedom to express oneself is to invite dis-ease.

It does not matter if we do not perceive ourselves as being 'creative' or 'artistic', although it would be interesting to know how many people who have psoriasis also experience some form of latent, suppressed or realised creative impulse?

Creative expression can occur in any form—overtly in free-form dance, privately in composing poetry or letters to friends, or as basically as using herbal preparations at home.

If competitiveness, success and materialism are more valuable than artistic expression, fluidity of thought or the decision to exist without subservience to a system of belief, we must be content in the knowledge that we are okay, it's all right to dance like this. I got a unique keratinocytic differentiation, baby! I can think this way if I want to. I can wear my disease in public; *they* haven't got it, and they need my genes if they think they're going to get it!

Relationships

Caring, love and compassion promote inner and outward reflecting states of health and well-being. Peace, love and harmony look nice as words on posters, too!

As a psoriatic, you could do with an empathetic companion to apply soothing lotions to the areas of your body you cannot reach, and with whom you could share your experiences, triumphs and troubles. It is of very great benefit to the emotional progress of healing to not only have the acceptance of 'self', but also to have another with whom to share the experience, the discoveries, and the joy of seeing the stuff recede and finally disappear.

Few things are better than the energies that bounce between two humans in direct, one to one contact and the interrelationship of conversation. The intimate presence of a person to person relationship is ideal, although even the phone line can suffice. It would be a shame if the only recourse we have is the Internet, as the electronic medium can be utterly soulless, and favours homogeneity at the expense of individuality. As interactive as it tries to be, and as far and wide and deep as its tentacles extend, the Internet was not developed to service this human need for intimate companionship or to enable its experience, and does not resonate with the natural laws and universal energy which are vital to human life.

Subtle energies

During the late nineteenth and into the early twentieth centuries, human-kind in its 'revolution' rediscovered the harmonic and electrical nature of existence. Following on from the Industrial Revolution, developments in communication technology and transportation helped open the collective mind to other realities. Interest in unseen forces, evidenced in Mesmerism, were rekindled at all levels of society alongside dissertations on reincarnation, 'the life beyond' and the possibility that we might not be alone in the universe. We know this because the 'élite' alongside the 'ordinary' person shared interest and experience, consequently news of it survived in the era's literature and has hung around in history. Material science flourished too, and geniuses with the insight of Nikola Tesla (1856–1943) forged immense discoveries which were precariously balanced on altruistic insight and materialistic realism (and duly vanished from mainstream recognition because of their altruism and therefore lack of recognition of the materialistic élitism).[6] With the interest created simultaneously in scientific development and 'spiritualistic' possibilities, there developed in the West an understanding of subtle energies.

Homeopathy

Homeopathy exhibits an innate understanding of the dynamic universal energy or life force that is present in all matter and which inspires real possibilities for self-healing. The modality works by administering the least possible medication to stimulate the body's autoimmune response.

Homeopathy, from *homeos*, 'similar', *pathos*, 'suffering', employs the principle of like treating like or, more specifically, the consequence of producing an effect which is similar to the suffering. The name for this subtle healing art was coined by Dr Samuel Hahnemann, who produced the first book on the subject in Germany in 1810. Hahnemann's discovery was a fortuitous accident and he always alluded to a number of people who revealed their understanding of its principles long before he did. These included Hippocrates, who stated that 'disease is produced by its similar ... fever is produced by what it suppresses, and suppressed by what it produces'. Paracelsus praised reasoning and experiment as the true sources of knowledge, and stated 'it is the similar which has to be compared with its similar ... comparison serves to reveal the secrets of healing'.

A trained physician and chemist, Hahnemann had renounced a career in medicine because of his dissatisfaction with the treatments he had been taught, and to avoid what he described as the risk of doing injury to his patients through the administration of such treatments as orthodox medicine then applied. Instead he practised chemistry and wrote and edited medical texts. Hahnemann was dismayed by the foolishness of the orthodox explanation provided for the action of Peruvian bark. This is our source of quinine, and the mainstream medical explanation was that it cured malaria because it was bitter. Dr Hahnemann decided to self-administer a series of doses of Peruvian bark. The result was his discovery that a drug which was known to cure a disease produced the symptoms of that disease in a healthy person. He experimented on other drugs in a similar fashion, and established that a substance that produces symptoms in a healthy person cures those symptoms in a sick person.

Hahnemann was also instrumental in the discovery of the law of the infinitesimal dose. At the level of dilution that homeopathic preparations are administered, there could remain barely a single molecule of the original substance—its healing effect is not the result of any chemical action by the drug. Instead, Hahnemann deduced the latent natural healing energy that is present in every substance in nature. He 'merely' hit upon the method of activating the life force—the energy that is in all matter—through his systematic processing.

In Britain, the Royal Homeopathic Hospital has been dispensing homeopathic preparations since 1849. During the nineteenth-century cholera epidemics in Europe, 40 per cent of patients treated with the contemporary orthodox medical response died, whereas only 9 per cent of homeopathy's patients succumbed.

There is another very important conclusion that can be drawn from homeopathy's ability to harness the energetic life force for healing. It is that the disorder on which the dynamic energy works is on the same plane, that is, the illness must be a derangement of the body's energy or life force. Acupuncture and acupressure share this principle of seeking to adjust the body's balance of energies by applying stimulation at predetermined sites, and thereby generating changes in the body's chemistry without chemical intervention.

A homeopath will provide specific remedies for the treatment of psoriasis, and respond to you wholistically in their assessment and careful deliberations.

Bach flower remedies

The 'essence', the 'life force', is present in all life. Like Hahnemann, the bacteriologist Dr Edward Bach lived at a time when the knowledge of these principles was being rediscovered. He pursued the enviable task of wandering the fields and valleys of England, Wales and continental Europe, discovering and collecting 38 different healing plants. He later extracted and preserved their healing essences. Dr Bach sought to prevent illness from manifesting in the physical body by altering the disharmonies of personality and emotional states, and restoring balance. Practitioners of this subtle healing art follow in Bach's footsteps by providing sympathetic treatment which helps remove negative emotions and thought forms while healing is being undertaken.

Traditional medicine

Traditional Chinese medicine understands and works with the same energy as does homeopathy, which in the oriental tradition is called *chi* or *qi* (also *qui*, *ki*), and *prana* in India. This energy is of the same source as the universal life force and has been known since very ancient times. Chi flows in the body along the meridians, and is reached via acupuncture or acupressure at key points (see *Figure 10*). It is essential that this energy flows properly, and it is influenced in this by its relationship with the body organs and various elements.[7]

CHINESE MEDICINE In Chinese medical philosophy, illness is a disturbance which indicates imbalance within the whole body system. Healing is approached by restoring balance and harmony to allow the body to heal itself. It will regain balance with the collaboration of the one who is ill, for stipulated dietary and habitual practices can either support or work against the treatment.

Acupuncture, herbal medicine and massage treat and work energetically with chi. Exercise programs such as Tai Chi and Qi Gung also work with and tone chi. Whether or not a belief in the effect of such treatment will influence its progress is a matter for the individual.

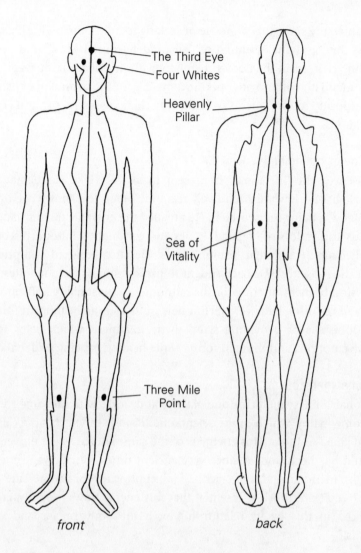

The Third Eye
Four Whites
Heavenly Pillar
Sea of Vitality
Three Mile Point
front
back

Figure 10: Examples, meridians and potent skin points

AYURVEDIC MEDICINE Ayurveda, 'the science of life' in the ancient Sanskrit, also embraces natural laws and wholistic philosophies; natural therapies are combined with individualised assessment, treatment and prevention. Lifestyle, diet and hygiene are all compatriots in good health, which is ultimately the ideal balance of energies in the body. The Ayurvedic or Vedic practitioner begins by determining the patient's constitution, which is a comprehensive profile. There are three main constitutions, or 'doshas', which include distinctions of physical type, activity style and personality. These energies (Air, Space, Fire, Water and Earth) are expressed in distinct combinations in the individual doshas, and treatment is developed to bring about this balance.

Detoxification, diet, breathing exercises, massage, meditation and sunbathing are employed to achieve a balance within the individual. Different foods and specific combinations of foods are determined according to the patient's dosha, with a particular emphasis on the taste of the food (bitter, sour, salty, pungent, sweet or astringent), the food's heat- or cold-producing qualities, and its consistency (oily or dry, light or heavy, liquid or solid). Eating a balance of all six tastes is recommended for people of all doshas, while animal proteins, processed foods, sugar and stimulants are to be avoided.

Ayurveda uses a comprehensive system to classify diseases, including the most important method, Origin. Diseases are also classified within the terms of the Sevenfold System, which allows for Genetic, Congenital, Constitutional, Traumatic, Seasonal, Infectious, Spiritual, and Natural divisions. Genetically determined diseases (*Adibalapravritta*) usually are attributed to defects in either the father's sperm or mother's ovum. In the case of obstinate skin diseases (*Kushta*), Ayurvedic medicine states that the reproductive elements of the mother or father were likely altered by unwholesome food, abnormal behaviour, addiction of any type, or stressful situations.

Underlying the Ayurvedic philosophy is the ability of the individual to achieve a healthy state of awareness through knowing one's self, and therefore being aware of the needs of one's body; the path to enlightenment is thus more easily achieved. At the very least, by knowing the dosha's needs, foods and practices which aggravate imbalance can be avoided, while actively living with the needs of the dosha firmly in mind will naturally result in cleansing and purifying practices, and therefore the prevention of disease. This is a specific and highly specialised system for which the practitioner's extensive knowledge is essential.

Acupressure

Acupressure and reflexology employ pressure directly from the good old human hand, fingers and thumbs, and work with the reflexes and the autonomic nervous system to release tension and ease pain. This counterpart of Swedish Massage, French Dō-In, and Japanese Shiatsu and Am-ma is a natural self-help therapy. It can be practised at any time, either solo or with the assistance of an empathetic companion.

Acupuncture and acupressure work on the premise that one's health is influenced by the flow of life force through the body in a system that shares a direct relationship with, but is physically distinct from, recognised neurological paths. The pressure which is applied through acupressure can be directed to either stimulate or sedate.

Treatment to specific points will gradually reveal a diminution of pain; in the Chinese tradition this signals recuperation and the dissipation of abnormal energies in the corresponding organ, and therefore the desired return to health.

Osteopathy

The skeleton and its supporting muscles and ligaments are subject to mechanical laws and the objects of stress and strain. Osteopathic medicine grew from the inspired mind of Dr Andrew Taylor Still, MD (1828–1917), a midwestern US frontier doctor, farmer, and Methodist.

Like his predecessor, Samuel Hahnemann, Andrew Still became dissatisfied with the medical status quo, and found the germ theory unacceptable. He observed an improvement in certain diseases when restricted muscles and skeletal joints were normalised through massage and manipulation.

Osteopathy is primarily manipulative treatment—osteopathy adjusts, nature heals. Naturopathic and osteopathic treatment together will incorporate diet, fasting, light, water and exercise, and psychological and manipulative adjustment. Osteopathic attention to one body area can improve the whole body condition.

It is osteopathy's concern to maintain the normal functioning of the body and all its systems. Osteopathy holds that dis-ease only occurs when all systems are not integrating or functioning as designed. This means that not only do the bones and muscles have to be okay, but so do the blood vessels and nerves, and all the visceral organs.

According to osteopathy, skin conditions usually indicate a breakdown of one of the body's other organs of elimination (liver, colon, lungs or kidneys) and that the skin has 'taken up the slack'. This is one area which the osteopath can check and correct. Due to the effect of emotions on the psoriatic condition, osteopathic treatment of the neck to relieve accumulated tension can also be beneficial.

Waxing and warping

Interest in homeopathy, Chinese medicine, acupuncture, Bach flower remedies, biochemic tissue salts and all other practices that understand and work with subtle energies waxes and wanes. Every now and then this interest finds new expression, as if the reality of the energies can't go away, as though to confirm and remind us of their direct relationship with us. Perhaps the message is being obscured by too much overhang from the Industrial Revolution way of doing things? What then of the new wave of alternatives?

Lanterns, pulses and beams

All matter is energy. All energy is vibration. All vibration is light. Sight, sound and feel are experiences of vibration.

What if thought, emotion and impulse were expressions of vibration?

The corporeal, the human body, as subtle and gross as it might or might not be, is an expression of energy, a clump of matter that vibrates at a predetermined rate. The human aura has been measured, and it has been found to vibrate at a rate higher than the solid mass of the physical body. Both the subtler auric field and the solid body share an interconnectedness with the energies that envelop, slice through and form the living matter that is the earth, including the electromagnetic fields that make up its physical form, its atmosphere and its subtler bodies and energetic matter. This energy is measured mathematically, and it can be expressed in musical notes.

Life force

The body reacts to light, colour and sound—expressions of the energy which is the life force in everything in this third dimension, and in those which are higher and lower. Energy is expressed in many forms including light, heat, sound and electricity.

Radiation is the process of energy when it is in motion and radiating away from its source, and is measured in wavelengths along a path called the electromagnetic spectrum. The term electromagnetic embraces electric and magnetic fields, which are distinct forms with an interconnectedness. Frequency is the term ascribed to the rate of fluctuation or oscillation of wavelengths within a single second.

Electric and magnetic fields can produce different effects on life forms. Of the two, magnetic fields pose the greater problem for human anatomy: the body will absorb magnetic fields in their entirety, and this affects the body's natural electrical balance.

Every living thing is in synchronisation with the earth's natural magnetic grid. Electrical and magnetic radiation factor in normal daily living, as electromagnetic frequencies are also emitted by technological devices as diverse as fluorescent lighting and communication antennae.

Vibrations of energy in the air constitute sound waves. The higher the pitch of sound, the greater the frequency, measured in cycles per second. Pitch is a property of sound and is measurable by frequency.

Electromagnetic frequencies (EMF) can be used to influence behaviour, and it has been shown in decades of studies that EMF exposure can trigger autoimmune diseases. Sound frequency can be applied to induce depression, agitation and rioting, confusion, anxiety and elation. Thus illness can be induced by electromagnetic energy bombardment. Responses to electromagnetic frequencies equivalent to the ambient background in a typical urban environment can produce temporary measurable changes in an individual's brain waves.[8] The levels, intensity and constancy of our body's exposure to radiation and frequencies of this nature can do harm to homeostasis, to say the least. Daily we are exposed to electromagnetic and other radiation from electrical power lines, microwaves, all manner of telecommunication devices, computers and TV. Consideration should be given to one's level of exposure.

Frequency response

Imagine being treated for illness with musical notes, harmonics or frequencies. In the 1930s, Dr Royal R. Rife developed an instrument which utilised electronics and the rule of resonance to treat illness and disease. He knew that a cell resonates with energy, and the instrument he developed was used to stimulate at this cellular level. This is intended to dissipate sick cells or destroy them completely. Rife's process became known as Radionics and has gathered its detractors.

There are various modalities and practitioners who understand and are applying basic principles of frequency in the treatment of disease. In Ohio in the USA, Sound Health Inc. has pioneered work with bio-acoustics. Heading up this research, Sharry Edwards MEd, has shown how some of the new pathogens, which have adopted a 'protective' protein sheath to enable them to lie disguised as a self cell and therefore safe from immune system attack, can be disarmed by the application of low-frequency sound.

Further to this work, it has been established that what the body does with nutritive compounds can be measured, predicted and described mathematically. This, as with any form of therapy which seeks to understand and apply the rules of universal frequency and harmony, offers appealing alternatives to any branch of medical science which takes the standpoint of denying the efficacy, or indeed refutes the existence of, such phenomena.[9]

Music's healing tones

Never mind its entertainment value, music in all of its expressions has the power to incite, lull, inspire … and heal. Just as the body reacts to light, colour and sound, so does it respond to music. However it is structured—to accompany a story-telling, propel a dance, or tease highly-tuned senses—music has the power to influence our health and emotions for better or worse.

The lover of one type of music who abhors another type is reacting to more than taste, be it refined or untrained—their vibrations are responding to the music's energy, its pulse, harmonic structures. Music can be used to incite a mob or enjoin a fervent patriotism, placate elevator-dwellers, or bring one to a state of ecstasy. An opera aficionado can be physically offended by rock because his or her energy (vibratory rate) is attuned to the 'classical' orchestral energy structures; a rapper can be repelled by symphonies because they are attuned to different energy patterns, be they 'good' or 'bad' for their personal electrical field. Neither is 'right' nor 'wrong'; both are experiencing emotional reactions to energy vibrations carried by and inherent in the musical energy and to which their biological and energetic selves are attuned through inclination and proclivity. Everyone is susceptible to the manipulation of these energetic preferences: they will buy clothing, drugs and consumer goods with equal commitment when the same frequencies are employed in the various media to conform with their tastes, or which are painstakingly manipulated to enhance them.

Consider also the effect of memory and emotion, and their interrelationship with music as an aural experience. How many times does a song remembered give rise to an emotional response, indeed a physical response—goose bumps, blushing, even tears? The emotion is triggered by a memory, which has been recalled by the music (vibration).

Music as an expression of the nature of civilisation and society of the past 2,000 years reflects the consciousness of the time and its people and their needs, according to Maria DeRungs, DMA, author of *The Healing Tones of Music*. The book describes the research and work of the Casa de Maria Research Centre, a music-therapy institute.

Music as medicine has been used since earliest recorded history. Sumerian art depicts beautiful instruments and their musicians, while it is known that the Egyptians and the Greeks used music for therapeutic purposes. Possibly these cultures had a better handle on the dynamic properties of the earth's natural magnetic grid than is currently understood. They might also have been aware that application of music and vibrational acoustics was therapeutically effective because it stimulated the human immune system, and consequently helped the body in its natural process of healing itself. It is known that music can affect physiological changes, such as stimulating the production of T cells.

The Tomatis Method, developed by Professor Alfred Tomatis whose methodology is practised in Europe, the USA and Australia, links impairment in auditory skills to learning and communication disorders, and general health problems such as fatigue and depression. The method cites the difference between hearing and listening, with the former being a passive sensory process of absorbing sound, and the latter a voluntary focusing on specific sounds. Tomatis uses specific music therapeutically, and suggests that new 'sonic drugs' such as loud rock music and the music played through the anti-personal portable stereo emit a low-pitch stimulus which can hypnotise and heighten bodily stimulation.[10]

The exploration of music as a possible adjunct to other therapies should not be overlooked.

Colour therapy
Colour is a property of light and is measurable by wavelengths. The application of colour to the body (chromotherapy), and the use of colour in visualisation and breathing, can be further useful ways of working with natural energies and frequencies. As with music, colour's use as therapy is nothing new.

In the practice of colour therapy, each of the seven visible colours of the spectrum is understood as having its own measurable wavelength, which in turn has a direct influence on an organ or aspect of the body system. The vital rhythm of an individual's unique frequency can be restored, and a balance between excesses and deficiencies obtained by the application of the appropriate colour(s). The visible colours of the spectrum are also directly associated with the chakras, or energy centres of the body.

Recourse to specific literature and/or practitioners in this field could be beneficial.

Electrical Nutrition
This is the title of a book by Denie and Shelley Hiestand, who make some very interesting claims about the value of food as it applies to the electrical body—indeed, they are adamant in their description of the entire process of nutrition as being an electrical one. Electrical malfunction precedes disease because of the food we eat, how we combine proteins and carbohydrates,

how our food is affected in its production and artificial processing, and indeed if our very choice of food is not in harmony with the natural electrical matrix (universal energy).

In many respects, the theory and practice inherent in their book, and the book you are reading now, share many characteristics and assertions, including the nature of vibrationary harmony and the 'biggest picture' (the Hiestands also speak out against the hijacking of the appellation 'traditional medicine' by orthodox allopathic medicine).

Psoriatics who have made the decision to address the intake of protein from animal sources, and have determined their metabolic type as the slow oxidiser who requires much less protein than a fast oxidiser, will be challenged by the theory and practice expounded in *Electrical Nutrition*. This theory holds that the best source of the electrical energy the body requires in its symbiotic relationship with the natural electrical matrix is animal meat; and further, that vegetarianism is anathema to optimum, vital health. Perhaps this is just another expression of the individuality and freedom of choice that are essential rights in pursuing health and well-being, and also points up— again—the value of working in collaboration with a gifted practitioner.

Personal power

We are fortunate to have the freedom to explore, write about and argue over the efficacies or otherwise of natural therapies, of revolutionary new and not-so-new ideas for healing, and the pros and cons of poisoning ourselves with foods and the way we live on and use the resources of this planet. Clearly there are those who are in the position to deny us our basic rights, and in this 'they' are ultimately more powerful by dint of their control of resources, money supply and the real estate. We should not give away any of our rights, the most basic of all being our entitlement to good health and well-being. Ultimately, how we achieve these is an individual matter. And it is in individuality that the key lies, together with the decision to act on behalf of our self, for our self.

Changing tune—being a hundredth monkey

Consider these facts.

- Life events stimulate the automatic release of naturally occurring neurochemicals (homologous drugs).
- The body in balance can supply painkillers and antibiotics without their creating side-effects.

- Synthetic drugs can harm brain patterns.
- The brain is a vital member of the immune system.

The treatment of degenerative disease with synthetic neurological or biological drugs arises from the development of analogues of chemicals which occur naturally within the body. Unlike the subtle, naturally occurring chemicals, synthesised drugs are non-selective and indiscriminate in their access to and effects on the body and brain.

Intrinsic to the processes occurring naturally in the body are the roles of neurotransmitters and receptor sites. These were identified by Candace Pert when working with Dr Solomon Snyder, at John Hopkins University in Baltimore, in 1973. The receptor, a brain site, will happily accommodate either a natural or a synthesised drug molecule. When the brain was found to possess receptors for morphine and heroin, early researchers wondered whether the body might produce its own versions of these substances, and whether addicts might merely be seeking instinctive supplementation of deficient or imbalanced neurochemicals. In 1975, two Scottish scientists, John Hughes and Hans Koesterlitz, confirmed the existence of natural body opiates, the endorphins.[11]

Importantly, ongoing research into neurotransmitters and neuropeptides identifies more and more of these that are present not only in the brain: neuropeptides and their receptors are found in the skin, stomach, intestines and heart. Monocytes, cells that form part of the immune system, travel through the bloodstream and interact with every cell in the body. Since they also carry receptors for brain chemicals, there is direct symbiosis between brain function (thought, intelligence) and immune system functions.

Many endorphins are associated with the experience of pain or pleasure and thus figure in the brain's internal reward system. When we engage in various activities, neurochemicals associated with pain or pleasure are released. For example, laughter and sex stimulate the energy of endorphins. As emotions of anger and fear, love and hate, are linked to brain functions, neurochemical reaction may be identified as influencing our reactions and behaviour, even thoughts, and vice versa. All animal brains contain the same DNA building blocks, the same patterns of neurochemicals; accordingly, animals feel emotions too. Superiority is made possible by the added human intellectual capacity that enables us to transcend our programming.

There is evidence of patients being willed to die under sentence of a disease having been proclaimed 'fatal'. Conversely, it is possible to reverse a degenerative pattern with the will to do so; the power of visualisation and conscious, decisive determination can be inherent in this. It could follow that hereditary predispositions might also be similarly overcome. An hereditary psoriatic imprint might thus be altered, even erased.

The 'hundredth monkey' in the heading above this section is borrowed from Ken Keyes Jnr's treatise in the public domain which in turn is derived from Lyall Watson's book *Lifetide*. The story is illuminating and provides a sense of empowerment to anyone who is willing to pursue or promote positive change, be it self-change or societal in its aspirations.

Lyall Watson tells of scientific observations on the Japanese island of Koshima in 1952. A tribe of Japanese macaques (*Macaca fuscata*) was fed sweet potatoes by the scientific team, but the monkeys found food that was dropped in the sand unpalatable. An eighteen-month-old female monkey named Imo discovered that washing her potatoes in a stream made the food more appetising. She taught the trick to her mother and her playmates, and in turn they taught their mothers. During the following six years, all of the young monkeys had learned to wash the sand from their potatoes, but only the adult animals which imitated their children learned the trick. Other adults continued to forsake the sandy potatoes. In the autumn of 1958, a certain number of Koshima island macaques were washing sweet potatoes—Keyes uses the number 99 to illustrate the point. He asks us to suppose that when the sun rose on a particular morning, 99 monkeys were washing their potatoes; by that evening almost all of the monkeys on the island were doing the same, which created an ideological breakthrough. Keyes repeats Lyall Watson's assertion that the practice was immediately observed amongst colonies of monkeys on other islands and amongst the group at Takasakiyama on the mainland. Sceptics decry the anecdote as a fabrication.

Whatever the reality, the importance of this tale lies in its modelling of the idea of quantum leaps in collective consciousness. It suggests that when a critical number achieves an awareness or makes a significant change of their own accord, the knowledge can be communicated from mind to mind, with the result of that change being spontaneously developed throughout the species. Ergo, when a critical number of people discover, create or adopt a new way, it becomes the conscious property of those people.

The hundredth monkey episode has a more recent counterpart in the life of migrating sperm whales off the east coast of Australia. In announcing the outcome of a five year study concluded in November 2000, whale researcher Michael Noad revealed that the herd had changed its tune. It is widely known that whale herds have their own 'call-signs'—communicative sounds that humans have come to liken to songs.

In the results of this study, which involved sound recordings of the herd on its annual migrations up and down the coast, it was discovered in 1998 that two out of 80 in the herd were using the different calls of whales from the west coast of Australia. These western whales had joined the eastern herd at some point in their Antarctic travels. Two migrations later, all 80 of the herd had adopted the new tunes. It was described as more of a 'revolution' than an 'evolution'. While this does not represent the quantum leap inherent in the Koshima monkey tale, it is nevertheless inspiring in its nature.[12]

Perhaps if sufficient numbers of psoriatics pursue detoxicating and healthier lifestyles, the quantum effect for us would be a gigantic physical and conscious upliftment, and an organic, genetic turning-point. Following this line of thought, if sufficient numbers of people could embrace the concept as a very real possibility, and consequently believe in their role in such a wild evolutionary process, we could be on the path to reversing hereditary indispositions to diseases such as psoriasis, indeed human biological imbalance in general. At the very least, the sum of human existence would be substantially uplifted, and you too would overcome psoriasis.

Appendix 1: Tables

Table 1: Irritant additives

These additives, of both natural and artificial origins, are known to irritate sensitive skin.

Number	Name
Colours	
102	Tartrazine
107	Yellow 2G
110	Sunset yellow FCF
122	Azorubine
123	Amaranth
124	Brilliant scarlet 4R
132	Indigo carmine
155	Brown HT
Preservatives	
210	Benzoic
211	Sodium benzoate
212	Potassium benzoate
213	Calcium benzoate
218	Methylparaben
221	Sodium sulphite
222	Sodium bisulphite
223	Sodium metabisulphite
224	Potassium metabisulphite
Antioxidant agents	
320	Butylated hydroxyanisole
321	Hydroxytoluene

Table 2: Skin, scalp and hair care

Creams	Oils	Lotions	Baths/ treatments
Allantoin	Almond	Aloe gel lotion	*Baths*
Goldenseal ointment	Apricot kernel	dilute with spring water*	Clay
Gotu kola ointment	Coconut butter and oil	Chlorophyll liquid	white for dry skin (soothing)
Hypericum cream	Jojoba	dilute with spring water*	green for oily skin (astringent)
Lanolin	Olive	Jojoba lotion	Oatmeal
Royal jelly	Sunflower		Cider vinegar (flaky dry skin)
Vitamin E cream	Sesame		
	Vitamins A and E		*Skin treatments*
	Wheat germ		Sea salt mixed with warm olive oil
		* At a ratio of 1:5 for the skin; 1:10 for the scalp	Almond meal mixed with warm apricot kernel oil

Recipe suggestions (see also *Chapter 6: On the Surface*)

SKIN MIX 1

4 tbsp aloe gel

1 tbsp warm coconut butter

(or 1 tbsp warm beeswax)

1 to 2 tbsp wheat germ oil

Blend aloe gel and coconut butter (or beeswax) and add wheat germ oil. Allow to cool, and store in a glass jar and refrigerate.

SKIN MIX 2

4 tbsp glycerine

1 to 2 tbsp lanolin (warmed)

2 to 3 tbsp vitamin E cream

(or 1 to 2 tbsp vitamin E oil)

Blend glycerine, lanolin and vitamin E cream (or oil). Allow to cool, and store in a glass jar and refrigerate.

HAIR AND SCALP MIX
250 ml liquid castile or base shampoo
50 ml aloe gel lotion or jojoba (wax/oil)
2 drops rosemary oil
Mix ingredients together and store in a glass jar.

Table 3: Amino acids

Many amino acids, with peptides and proteins, are synergists that increase the effectiveness of other antioxidants. They are made available by the digestion of any food containing protein.

Sources which can be regarded as possible 'triggers' for psoriatics are *italicised*.

The best natural sources of nutrients are listed in a general order, rather than from highest to lowest.

Sources	Functions
Alanine	
AFA, spirulina Most protein sources Wheat germ *Cottage cheese* *Pork*	Strengthens cell walls Competes with taurine transport Regulates glucose metabolism
Arginine	
AFA *Chicken* Almonds, pecans, cashews Peas Garlic Ginseng Whole wheat	Heals tissue A detoxifier Stimulates growth hormone in the pituitary gland, and T-lymphocyte production Figures in collagen and elastin synthesis Enhances protein synthesis Inhibits cellular proliferation Facilitates seminal fluid (80 per cent of which is arginine)
Aspartic acid	
AFA, spirulina Avocado Asparagus Sprouts	Metabolises carbohydrates to produce cellular energy

(Amino acids)

Sources	Functions
Carnitine	
Animal foods Spirulina, AFA	Needed for muscle functions Targets muscles and hair protein Made from lysine and methionine
Choline	
Lecithin, egg yolk *Organ and muscle meats* Legumes, nuts Comfrey	Necessary for the production of the neurotransmitter acetylcholine An important co-enzyme in metabolism A chemical detoxifier
Cysteine	
AFA, spirulina Eggs Fish, sardines Chicken *Beef, liver* *Cottage cheese, milk*	Stabilises blood sugar An antioxidant (with the ability to chelate and expel heavy metals from the system) Metabolises carbohydrates Needed for the optimum utilisation of B_6
Glutamine	
AFA, spirulina Rolled oats Cottage and ricotta cheese *Meats* Fish	Can become an essential amino acid in the presence of extreme stress or illness Brain fuel, needed for memory Helps speed the healing of peptic ulcers
Glutathione	
Most protein sources Garlic	An antioxidant Detoxifies the body of heavy metals Synergistic with selenium Targets the liver Inhibits the enzyme lipoxygenase which is implicated in psoriasis

(Amino acids)

Sources	Functions
Glycine	
AFA, spirulina Most protein sources	Promotes energy oxygen use in the cells and liver detoxification Active in the synthesis of bile salts and nucleic acids A constituent of collagen
Histidine	
AFA Fish Eggs *Meats* Wheat germ Cottage cheese Soybeans	Strengthens the nerve relays Targets the auditory organ A precursor to histamine Stimulates stomach acid secretion
Isoleucine	
AFA, spirulina Most protein sources Chick peas, lentils Almonds Pumpkin, sunflower, sesame seeds	Demand is increased by liver disease and renal dysfunction Active in haemoglobin production
Leucine	
AFA, spirulina Most protein sources Brazil nuts	Promotes wound healing
Lysine	
AFA, spirulina Most protein sources Comfrey leaf Brewer's yeast Bean sprouts Oats Onions	An important agent in fat metabolism Facilitates calcium absorption A constituent of collagen and elastin Enhances concentration

(Amino acids)

Sources	Functions
Methionine	
AFA, spirulina *Dairy products* *Meat* *Poultry*	Targets the memory A chelator, i.e. combines with heavy metals (lead, mercury) and eliminates them from the body
Phenylalanine	
AFA, spirulina *Meat* *Cheese*	Necessary for mental alertness (brain adrenalin) Requires adequate vitamin C for proper metabolism The parent substance of tyrosine and therefore essential for normal thyroid gland function
Proline	
AFA, spirulina Most protein sources Wheat germ	A precursor of glutamic acid A principal amino acid in connective tissue proteins A constituent of collagen and elastin
Serine	
AFA, spirulina Most protein sources Wheat germ	Protects fatty sheaths of nerve fibres (the myelin sheath) An additive to commercial cosmetics for its natural moisturising properties
Taurine	
Animal meats Eggs Fish *Shellfish* *Milk*	A neurotransmitter Stimulates the synthesis of growth hormone Assists with bile synthesis and heart function Synthesises with zinc Influences insulin and blood sugar levels Normalises the balance of other amino acids
Threonine	
AFA, spirulina *Animal protein* *Dairy products* Eggs Pulses Deficient in grains	Prevents excess liver fat Promotes digestive and intestinal tract functions An immune system stimulant Maintains connective tissue

(Amino acids)

Sources	Functions
Tryptophan	
AFA, spirulina *Milk* *Cottage cheese* Lentils, soybeans Fish *Beef* *Peanuts* Sesame, pumpkin seeds	Converts in the brain to serotonin Necessary for the synthesis of vitamin B_3 Essential for normal sleep patterns (deficiencies can underlie poor skin tone, brittle nails, insomnia, depression and mental disturbance) Stimulates liver protein synthesis
Tyrosine	
AFA, spirulina *Meat* *Cheese* Soybeans Almonds Eggs Fish	An anti-depressant The amino acid needed by the thyroid gland Slows ageing Targets skin, hair and mental health Alleviates hay fever and grass allergies
Valine	
AFA, spirulina *Beef, lamb* *Chicken*, fish *Cottage cheese* Nuts Chick peas, lima beans, soybeans *Mushrooms*	Necessary for the normalisation of the body's nitrogen balance Essential for neural and mental function, and muscle coordination

Table 4: Enzymes and other nutrients

Enzymes dismantle and convert remaining nutrients into simpler substances which the body can use—proteins into amino acids; fats into fatty acids; carbohydrates into glucose.

Peeling, cooking, pasteurising, refining and preserving largely destroy enzymes in food.

Sources which can be regarded as possible 'triggers' for psoriatics are *italicised*.

The best natural sources of nutrients are listed in a general order, rather than from highest to lowest.

Enzyme/ nutrient	Sources	Functions and comments
Bromelain	Pineapple	A digestive enzyme
Dietary fibre	Psyllium husks, bran Linseed Celery, leafy greens, root vegetables Apples, bananas Legumes, nuts, seeds Comfrey Agar, some sea vegetables	Facilitates healthy digestion Over-productive hostile bacteria will decompose fibre causing it to fail before it has the chance to stimulate bowel movement Destroyed in cereal grains by food processing and refining methods

Enzyme/ nutrient	Sources	Functions and comments
Germanium	Aloe vera, comfrey Ginseng Garlic	Enriches the body's oxygen supply An important immune system ally in its activation of macrophages
Glucosamine	Synthesised in the body from glucose	A major precursor to the synthesis of mucopolysaccharides A component of the stomach's protective mucous lining
Lactobacillus acidophilus	*Yoghurt*	Replenishes beneficial bacteria in the intestines (especially necessary following a course of antibiotics)
Lecithin	Unrefined cold-pressed vegetable oils Egg yolk Nuts, seeds Soybeans	A complete combination of phospholipids, phosphoric acid, choline, inositol and methionine Aids the transportation of fats throughout the body Mobilises and disperses fat and cholesterol deposits With cholesterol, is essential in the production of bile
Mucopoly-saccharides	Aloe vera, comfrey Slippery elm, ginseng Oatmeal, wheat germ Oysters, *shellfish*	A basic unit of carbohydrate, with glucose being the most common Found in all body tissues and fluids Provides a protective barrier to mucous membranes Promotes tissue regeneration Depleted by cortisone

Table 5: Herbs

SURFACE ←→ INTERNAL

Skin cleansing and stimulating	Skin cell growth	Reducing skin inflammation	Digestive aids	Digestive canal lubricants (demulcents)	Tonics and blood purifiers	Immune system
Aloe vera	Barberry	Boswellia	Alfalfa	Arrowroot	Barberry	Allspice
Chamomile	Goldenseal	Chamomile	Allspice	Comfrey	Burdock	Cat's claw
Goa	Gotu kola	Comfrey	Aloe vera	Iceland moss	Dandelion	Cloves
Goldenseal	Oregon grape	Hypericum (St John's wort)	Barberry	Irish moss	Ginseng	Ginseng
Rosemary		Milk thistle	Basil	Liquorice root	Horseradish	Goldenseal
Soap tree		Red clover	Comfrey	Marshmallow	Milk thistle	Horseradish
Southernwood		Sage	Coriander	Slippery elm	Olive leaf	Milk thistle
Water betony		Yellow dock	Lemongrass		Oregano	Oregano
			Mullein		Parsley	Parsley
			Peppermint		Red clover	Red clover
			Rosemary		Rosemary	Rosemary
			Slippery elm		Sage	Sarsaparilla
					Sarsaparilla	Sage
					Thyme	Thyme
					Yarrow	

Table 6: Vitamins and essential nutrients

Sources which can be regarded as possible 'triggers' for psoriatics are *italicised*.

The best natural sources of nutrients are listed in a general order, rather than from highest to lowest.

(Vitamins and essential nutrients)

Vitamin/ nutrient	Sources	Depleted by	Assists / comments	Roles	Synergises with	Targets
A	Fish liver oils (highest in cod, salmon and halibut) Apricots, carrots (yellow fruits and vegetables) Sweet potato, *tomatoes,* asparagus, broccoli, cabbage Eggs *Liver, beef, veal* *Dairy products, feta cheese*	Exposure to heat and light Alcohol Coffee Smoking Pesticides Oral contraceptives	Growth and repair of cells and membranes Synthesis of mucopolysaccharides	Fights bacteria and infection Maintains healthy tissues, and intestinal and mucosal linings	B_2, B_3, B_{12} C E Calcium Iodine Zinc Thyroxine Testosterone	Skin Eyes Hair and scalp Gums Joints Glands Intestine

(Vitamins and essential nutrients)

Vitamin/ nutrient	Sources	Depleted by	Assists / comments	Roles	Synergises with	Targets
B$_1$	Brewer's yeast, molasses *Liver, poultry* Fish, egg yolk Whole grains and seeds, nuts Zucchini, asparagus, cabbage, *peppers, peas, tomatoes,* sprouts Pulses, legumes Rice, bran Kelp (seaweed), AFA, spirulina	Cooking, roasting and milling Sugar	Carbohydrate metabolism Food assimilation and digestion Efficient waste exchange Brain function Nerve cell nutrition Gastrointestinal health	Energy producer	All other B vitamins Choline Magnesium Manganese Molybdenum Phosphate	Liver Kidneys Intestinal muscle tone Digestive system Skin Hair Eyes Brain Heart

(Vitamins and essential nutrients)

Vitamin/ nutrient	Sources	Depleted by	Assists / comments	Roles	Synergises with	Targets
B₂	Avocado Eggs, *chicken* *Mushrooms*, green leafy vegetables Wholegrain cereals Currants, almonds *Tomatoes, chillies* Bean sprouts, bamboo shoots Brewer's yeast Legumes, lentils Mackerel Kelp (seaweed), AFA, spirulina *Organ meats* *Cottage cheese, dairy foods*	Exposure to heat and light Food processing Oral contraceptives Baking powder	Fat, carbohydrate and protein metabolism Antibody formation Red blood cell formation Cell respiration	Repairs and maintains healthy skin Regulates body acidity Energy producer	A All Bs Biotin Magnesium Copper Iron Molybdenum Hydrochloric acid	Skin Hair Nails Eyes Immune system Digestive system

(Vitamins and essential nutrients)

Vitamin/ nutrient	Sources	Depleted by	Assists / comments	Roles	Synergises with	Targets
B$_3$	Tuna, salmon, sardines, mackerel *Chicken, turkey* *Mushrooms, asparagus, cabbage, beets* Almonds, sunflower seeds, *peanuts* Rice bran *Milk* Brewer's yeast Kelp (seaweed)	Ethylene oxide (used to ripen fruit) results in 50% loss	Fat, carbohydrate and protein metabolism Detoxification	Maintains healthy skin and hair Aids digestive system Balances blood sugar Lowers blood cholesterol Stimulates gastric and bile secretion Decreases the effects of hallucinogens	B$_1$, B$_2$, B$_6$, B$_{12}$ Folic acid Zinc Copper Chromium Iron Magnesium Potassium Molybdenum Methionine Selenium Leucine Tryptophan	Skin Gastrointestinal tract Liver Kidneys Heart Muscle Brain Central nervous system

(Vitamins and essential nutrients)

Vitamin/ nutrient	Sources	Depleted by	Assists / comments	Roles	Synergises with	Targets
B5	*Organ meats* Strawberries, cherries Celery, *mushrooms,* green vegetables Brewer's yeast, egg yolk Royal jelly Legumes, whole grains, *peanuts,* brown rice, wheat germ Salmon, kelp (seaweed), AFA, spirulina	Heat Food processing Milling Stress Alcohol Coffee Tea	The formation of some fat and the release of energy from carbohydrates, fats and proteins Maintenance of healthy mucosal lining Conversion of uric acid into urea and ammonia	Stimulates adrenal glands Increases production of cortisone and other adrenal hormones Maintains healthy digestive tract Improves body's resistance to stress Stimulates glutathione levels	C Bs Biotin Folic acid Iron Chromium Zinc Phosphate Methionine Cysteine	All tissues Skin Hair and scalp Nerves Glands

(*Vitamins and essential nutrients*)

Vitamin/ nutrient	Sources	Depleted by	Assists / comments	Roles	Synergises with	Targets
B$_6$	Oatmeal, wheat germ *Offal* Red kidney beans, lentils, legumes Seeds, *peanuts*, walnuts Egg yolk, *chicken* Salmon, tuna, mackerel Watercress, *peppers*, avocado, squash, broccoli, brussels sprouts, asparagus, onions Bananas Molasses Kelp (seaweed), AFA, spirulina	Exposure to heat and light Freezing Oral contraceptives High protein diet Food processing	Amino acid synthesis Carbohydrate, fat and protein metabolism Production of hydrochloric acid Production of red blood cells	Activates the release of glycogen from the liver and muscles Assists muscle energy Promotes normal nervous and musculo-skeletal systems Helps control allergic reactions Increases dopamine in the brain Assists antibody formation Maintains sodium, phosphorus and potassium balance Assists brain function and hormone production	All Bs C Biotin Iron Chromium Potassium Zinc Magnesium Copper Dolomite Phosphate Sodium	Skin Nails Tongue Lips Nervous tissue Liver Lymph nodes Muscle tissue Circulatory system

(Vitamins and essential nutrients)

Vitamin/ nutrient	Sources	Depleted by	Assists / comments	Roles	Synergises with	Targets
B$_{12}$	Freshwater algae, kelp (seaweed)	Heat	Normal blood cell formation and oxidation	Synthesises folic acid and aids the conversion of vitamin A	A	Skin
	Liver, kidney, brains, muscle meats, pork	Light	Biosynthesisor nucleic acids, protein and blood cells	Maintains gut, epithelial and mucosal cells	B$_1$, B$_5$	Hair
	Oysters, sardines, salmon, herring	Alkalines	Carotene absorption	Maintains normal bone marrow and a healthy nervous system	C	Bones
	Eggs	Acids		Metabolises carbohydrates, fats and proteins	E	Central nervous system
	Dairy products				Biotin	Kidneys
	Mushrooms				Folic acid	Heart
	Comfrey				Iron	Muscle
					Calcium	Stomach
					Cobalt	
					Copper	
					Methionine	
					Phosphate	

(Vitamins and essential nutrients)

Vitamin/ nutrient	Sources	Depleted by	Assists / comments	Roles	Synergises with	Targets
Bioflavenoids	Vegetable and fruit skins Citrus fruits (particularly white flesh), blackcurrants, plums, grapes, cherries, papaya, melon, berries, rosehips Onions, garlic, *tomatoes*, broccoli, cucumber Buckwheat *Tea, red wine*	Free radicals	Helps build capillary strength A modulator of metabolic enzymes Readily absorbed via the gastrointestinal tract into the bloodstream	Antioxidants	B$_6$ C E Zinc Tyrosine	Skin Gastrointestinal tract Musculo-skeletal system Vascular system

(Vitamins and essential nutrients)

Vitamin/ nutrient	Sources	Depleted by	Assists / comments	Roles	Synergises with	Targets
Biotin	Bacterial synthesis in the gut

Egg yolk, *liver, organ meats*

Brewer's yeast, whole grains, sweet corn, unpolished rice, cereals, soybeans, legumes, almonds

Peanuts

Sardines, oysters, AFA, spirulina

Cauliflower, lettuce, peas, bean sprouts

Grapefruit, watermelon | Acids and alkalis

Grain processing

Alcohol

Coffee

Raw egg white

Fried food

Rancid fats

Choline | Carbohydrate, fat and protein metabolism

Utilisation of other B group vitamins and pantothenic acid | Maintains skin, hair and sebaceous glands

Aids cell growth

Aids liver function

Essential for the synthesis of niacin | All Bs

Folic acid

Iron

Manganese

Magnesium

Pantothenic acid

Testosterone | Skin

Hair

Nervous tissue

Male genitalia

Bone marrow

Liver

Kidney |

(*Vitamins and essential nutrients*)

Vitamin/ nutrient	Sources	Depleted by	Assists / comments	Roles	Synergises with	Targets
C	*Chillies, pimientos, peppers, potatoes, red cabbage, tomatoes,* alfalfa seeds, sprouts, kale, mustard, dandelion and watercress greens, parsley Citrus fruits, pineapple, berries, blackcurrants, guava, acerola cherry, Kiwi fruit, melons, papaya, mangoes, rosehips *Liver*	Heat Light Acids and alkalis Food processing Stress Pollution Fried food Chopping Salting Drying	Wound healing, fractures and the formation of scar tissue An antioxidant and antibiotic Antiviral and antibacterial Essential to the metabolic process Protects the oxidation of iron in the intestine	Strengthens the immune system Activates enzymes and folic acid Strengthens blood vessels Assists red blood cell development Regulates metabolism of cholesterol Maintains collagen Aids resistance to stress	Bioflavenoids A B_5, B_6, B_{12} E Folate Calcium Iron Magnesium Manganese Selenium Zinc Lysine Methionine	Skin Adrenal cortex Pituitary gland Reproductive glands Connective tissue Bone Liver Teeth Gums

(Vitamins and essential nutrients)

Vitamin/ nutrient	Sources	Depleted by	Assists / comments	Roles	Synergises with	Targets
Choline	Lecithin, brewer's yeast, wheat germ Whole grains *Liver*, fish Beans, soybeans, legumes *Peanuts* Citrus AFA *Milk*, egg yolk	Alcohol Oral contraceptives	Chemical detoxification Transmission of nerve impulses Stronger capillary walls (reduces high blood pressure) A co-enzyme in metabolism	Assists utilisation of fats and cholesterol Synthesises lecithin	B_5, B_{12} Folic acid Lecithin Methionine Inositol Ethanolamine	Liver Kidneys Heart Central nervous system Lungs

(Vitamins and essential nutrients)

Vitamin/ nutrient	Sources	Depleted by	Assists / comments	Roles	Synergises with	Targets
D	Fish liver oils (tuna, cod, herring, halibut) Salmon, sardines, pilchards, eel, oysters Kelp (seaweed) Sprouted seeds *Organ meats* *Dairy products,* egg yolk Bone meal	Light Lack of sunlight Fried food	A stable nervous system Normal heart action	Promotes the absorption and utilisation of calcium and phosphorus Regulates the immune system Assists bone formation	Sunlight B_3 K Calcium Magnesium Manganese Phosphorus Sodium Boron Silica Parathyroid hormone	Skin Hair Teeth Bones Joints Muscle Kidney Intestine Liver Pancreas Brain

(Vitamins and essential nutrients)

Vitamin/ nutrient	Sources	Depleted by	Assists / comments	Roles	Synergises with	Targets
E	Sunflower, sesame and watermelon seeds Eggs, *beef* Brown rice, whole grains, wheat germ and wheat germ oil, soybean and safflower oil, corn oil unrefined, oatmeal, bran Tuna, salmon, sardines, oysters, kelp (seaweed), AFA, spirulina Leafy vegetables, broccoli, cauliflower, sweet potato, peas Nuts (Brazil, almonds, pecans, hazelnut, walnuts, *peanuts*)	Heat Light Alkalis Milling Pollution Oral contraceptives Refined or processed fats and oils Chlorine in drinking water Rancid oil or fat Copper and iron cooking utensils	Wound healing Cellular respiration Fertility An antioxidant A diuretic	Protects fat-soluble vitamins Protects red blood cells Lowers blood pressure Aids nourishment to the cells Inhibits blood coagulation Aids gastro-intestinal function Promotes immune system function Promotes a healthy muscular system	A B_2, B_6, B_{12} C K Folic acid Selenium Copper Manganese Zinc Cysteine	Skin Eyes Muscles Glands Intestines Heart Vascular system

(Vitamins and essential nutrients)

Vitamin/ nutrient	Sources	Depleted by	Assists / comments	Roles	Synergises with	Targets
Essential fatty acids	Fish, wheat germ, evening primrose, soybean, walnut, rapeseed, corn, linseed, sesame and sunflower oils AFA, spirulina, seaweed Lecithin, tofu, *chicken, game,* eggs, butter	Hydrogenation Light Heat	Fat dissolving Visual function Vitamin D absorption Carotene conversion to vitamin A	Maintains cellular membrane structure Promotes blood coagulation Regulates inflammation reactions	A B_3, B_6 Bioflavenoids E Magnesium Zinc Selenium Methionine	Skin Blood Heart Arteries Nerves Growth Eyes Organs Muscle

(Vitamins and essential nutrients)

Vitamin/ nutrient	Sources	Depleted by	Assists / comments	Roles	Synergises with	Targets
Folic acid	Avocado, sprouts, spinach, asparagus, broccoli, lettuce, *mushrooms*, root vegetables Oranges, strawberries Walnuts, cashews, hazelnuts, beans, lentils, soybeans, rice, brewer's yeast *Milk, eggs* Oysters, kelp, AFA, spirulina, salmon *Organ meats*	Exposure to heat and light Food processing Oral contraceptives Smoking	Healing intestinal disturbances and skin disorders An essential co-enzyme in metabolism— aids metabolism of proteins necessary for growth and cell division Stimulates production of hydrochloric acid Treats deficient absorption of nutrients from the intestine	Red blood cell formation Aids brain functions	B_3, B_5, B_{12} C E Biotin Methionine Copper Iron Zinc Magnesium	Liver Bone marrow Lymph nodes Kidneys

(Vitamins and essential nutrients)

Vitamin/ nutrient	Sources	Depleted by	Assists / comments	Roles	Synergises with	Targets
Inositol	Lecithin, brewer's yeast Seeds, beans, chick peas, brown rice, nuts, whole grains, oatmeal, lentils Fruits, cantaloupe *Tomatoes*, vegetables Corn, corn oil, soya flour, molasses *Milk, eggs, fish, beef, veal, pork, liver*	Antibiotics Freezing Canning Alcohol Tea Coffee Oral contraceptives Diuretics Phytates	Saturated fat absorption from the intestine Cell growth Formation of the nerve sheath Liver function Myelin synthesis Zinc absorption Formation of prothrombin (blood coagulant) in the liver	Fat-dissolving Reduces blood cholesterol Maintains healthy hair A component of cell membranes	B_3, B_6 Biotin Choline Folic acid EPA Pantothenic acid	Liver Alimentary canal Skin Hair Eyes Brain Spinal cord

(Vitamins and essential nutrients)

Vitamin/ nutrient	Sources	Depleted by	Assists / comments	Roles	Synergises with	Targets
K	Bacterial synthesis in the gut Lecithin, egg yolk *Liver, pork* Kelp Green plants and leafy green vegetables, cauliflower, asparagus, *potatoes*, watercress Lemongrass, alfalfa *Yoghurt*, kefir and acidophilus milk (assist the body with manufacturing sufficient amounts) Molasses Safflower oil Oats, whole wheat, brown rice, soybeans Fish liver oils Dates Tahini Almonds, cashews	Light Alkalis Fats Industrial air pollution Mineral oil Radiation X-rays Aspirin Antibiotics Sulphur drugs Phenobarbitol Salicylates	Liver function Calcium metabolism Bone mineralisation Growth Some produced by bacteria in healthy intestines	Controls blood clotting— essential for the production of prothrombin A natural food preservative	A B_3, B_6 C E Manganese Co-enzyme Q_{10}	Liver Vascular system

Table 7: Minerals

Sources which can be regarded as possible 'triggers' for psoriatics are *italicised*.

The best natural sources are listed in a general order, rather than from highest to lowest.

(Minerals)

Mineral	Sources	Assists / maintains	Synergises with
Boron	AFA Leafy vegetables, greens, parsnips, carrots, beetroot Almonds, hazelnuts Apples, pears, prunes, raisins Soy milk *Peanut butter*	Efficient absorption of calcium Activation of vitamin D in a synergistic relationship with the kidneys	B₂ D Magnesium

(Minerals)

Mineral	Sources	Assists/ maintains	Synergises with
Calcium	Almonds, pumpkin seeds	Regulation of hormone secretion	A
	Sardines, salmon, oysters, *shellfish*	Regulation of cell division and passage of nutrients in and out of the cell wall	C
	Sea vegetables, AFA, spirulina	Maintains nerve transmission	D
	Oats, corn	Maintains muscle growth and contraction	K
	Egg yolk	Utilisation of iron	Boron
	Yoghurt, buttermilk, ricotta cheese, Parmesan cheese, whey, goat's milk, *Swiss cheese, Cheddar cheese*	Activates and regulates digestive enzymes	Magnesium
	Soybeans, tofu	Maintains the blood's alkaline, acid and electrolyte balance	Phosphorus
	Molasses, brewer's yeast	*Noteworthy*	Lysine
	Asparagus, broccoli, green leafy vegetables, globe artichokes, okra, parsley, mustard greens	Essential for healthy teeth and bones	Arginine
	Figs, prunes	Absorbed in the duodenum and upper jejunum	
	Carob	Absorption ends in the lower intestinal tract when the food content becomes alkaline	
	Dolomite, bone meal	Destroyed by alcohol, lack of hydrochloric acid and exercise, caffeine, stress, and hormonal imbalances	
		Excessive protein consumption causes loss of calcium from the bones	
		Oxalic acid in chocolate, cocoa, rhubarb and spinach can inhibit calcium absorption	
		Phytates, naturally occurring chemicals, will also interfere with calcium absorption	

(Minerals)

Mineral	Sources	Assists/ maintains	Synergises with
Copper	Nuts (Brazil, walnuts, cashews, *peanuts*) Beans Oysters, *shellfish, crustaceans* AFA, spirulina Prunes *Lamb, pork, organ meats* Eggs, *yoghurt* *Poultry* Molasses Avocado, *mushrooms* Whole grains, oatmeal, barley Lentils Sunflower seeds, wheat germ Garlic	Maintenance of skin, bone and nerve functions Protein metabolism The conversion of tyrosine into melanin Vitamin C oxidisation Formulation of elastin in conjunction with vitamin C Melanin, myelin, collagen and elastin synthesis Regulation of iron metabolism ***Noteworthy*** Chief component of elastic connective tissue throughout the body Preserves membrane strength Protects against free radicals Absorbed in the stomach and small intestine A constituent of an antioxidant enzyme implicated in inflammatory reactions (e.g. rheumatoid arthritis)	B_2, B_6, B_{12} Iron Manganese Folic acid Amino acids

(Minerals)

Mineral	Sources	Assists/ maintains	Synergises with
Iodine	Kelp and sea vegetables in general	Maintenance of healthy skin and hair	B complex
	White deepwater fish, oysters	Thyroid hormone synthesis	C
	Sunflower and sesame seeds	Cell division	Copper
	Mushrooms, spinach, Swiss chard, garlic	Carotene conversion to vitamin A	Magnesium
	Iodised salt	Physical and mental development	Zinc
	Dairy products, eggs	***Noteworthy***	Tyrosine
	Lima beans, soybeans	Provision is very low or absent in refined foods	
		Absorbed through all of the gastrointestinal tract	
		Iodine can irritate acne	

(Minerals)

Mineral	Sources	Assists / maintains	Synergises with
Iron	AFA, spirulina, kelp	Transportation of oxygen and carbon dioxide to and from cells	A
	White deepwater fish, oysters, clams, mussels, salmon	Skin and nail formation	B complex
	Organ meats, pork	Energy production	C
	Egg yolk, *poultry*	Synthesis of haemoglobin and collagen	E
	Wheat germ, bulgur wheat, brown rice, oats	Neurotransmitter synthesis	Calcium
	Molasses, brewer's yeast, tahini	Strong immune system	Folic acid
	Cherry juice, apricots, strawberries, prunes, raisins, dates	Resistance to stress	Copper
	Leafy green vegetables, avocado, pumpkin, parsley		Manganese
	Soybeans, chick peas, beans	*Noteworthy*	Molybdenum
	Pine nuts, Brazil nuts, cashews, almonds, walnuts, pecans, sunflower and pumpkin seeds	Absorbed through the duodenum, stomach and upper jejunum	Phosphorus
			Selenium
			Citrate
			Lysine
			Hydrochloric acid
			Histidine

(Minerals)

Mineral	Sources	Assists / maintains	Synergises with
Magnesium	AFA, spirulina, seafood Almonds, cashews Lima beans, lentils, soybeans, tofu Brewer's yeast, bone meal, molasses, wholegrain cereals Avocado, parsnips, corn, garlic Figs, raisins, black grapes, black cherries, apples, stone fruit, grapefruit	Lecithin production Many metabolic processes, including energy production of protein, glucose Other minerals' metabolism and absorption Nerve and muscle function Cell formation Bone growth Body temperature regulation Concentration *Noteworthy* Necessary for the production of calcium and vitamin C Absorbed through the duodenum and ileum Substantial loss through the milling process Destroyed by large amounts of calcium in milk products, proteins and fats	B_1 B_6 C D Potassium

(*Minerals*)

Mineral	Sources	Assists / maintains	Synergises with
Manganese	AFA, spirulina	Activation of more than 20 enzymes—an enzyme activator and co-factor in lipid and carbohydrate metabolism	B$_1$
	Sunflower seeds		C
	Whole grains, corn	Synthesis of cholesterol, mucopolysaccharides, glutamine and thyroxine	E
	Legumes, dried peas, kidney beans		K
	Walnuts, pecans, almonds	A healthy immune system	Biotin
	Avocado, spinach, green vegetables, okra	Synthesis and reproduction of red blood cells	Choline
	Egg yolk	Utilisation of thiamine and vitamin E	Copper
	Olives	Insulin production	Iron
	Blueberries, raspberries, strawberries, grapes, pineapple, coconut	Healthy nerves and brain functions	Zinc
	Kelp (seaweed)	*Noteworthy*	
	Liver	Stabilises blood sugar	
		Absorbed in the small intestinal tract	
		40% of the manganese ingested is absorbed by the body	
		Iron competes with manganese absorption	
		Lost in the milling process	
		Destroyed by alcohol, antibiotics and refined foods	

(Minerals)

Mineral	Sources	Assists / maintains	Synergises with
Molybdenum	Legumes, soybeans Whole grain cereals, wheat germ Sunflower seeds Molasses Dark green leafy vegetables AFA *Liver, kidney* *Butter*	The mobilisation of iron from the liver Fat, iron and copper metabolism	Proteins, including amino acids which contain sulphur

(Minerals)

Mineral	Sources	Assists / maintains	Synergises with
Phosphorus	AFA, spirulina Sesame seeds Almonds, cashews Dried fruit Oatmeal Tuna, salmon, sardines *Dairy products* *Organ meats* Garlic Chick peas, legumes *Poultry*, eggs Brewer's yeast	Digestion of niacin and riboflavin Utilisation of carbohydrates, fats and proteins for energy production Activation of most B vitamins Kidney function Nerve impulse transference, and maintenance of healthy nerves and mental activity Stimulates muscle contractions Formulation and maintenance of bones and teeth (with calcium) Muscle tissue building pH balance Maintenance of the constant composition of body fluids *Noteworthy* A component of DNA, RNA, phosphoproteins and phospholipids (e.g. cholesterol) Absorbed through the duodenum, jejunum and ileum Affected by excessive iron or magnesium	B complex D Calcium Potassium

(Minerals)

Mineral	Sources	Assists / maintains	Synergises with
Potassium	AFA, spirulina Sardines, herrings, salmon, red snapper, sea vegetables All vegetables, *potatoes* (especially the skin), beet greens, avocado Apricots, bananas, citrus, dates, figs, raisins, prunes Almonds, cashews, pecans Brewer's yeast, brown rice, molasses *Milk*, yoghurt Mint leaves	Healthy skin Protein and carbohydrate metabolism, synthesis and hydration Kidney elimination and gut movements Regulation of water balance within the body Stable blood pressure and osmotic pressure Transference of nutrients to cells Normalisation of the heartbeat in conjunction with sodium Enzyme reaction and electrolyte balance ***Noteworthy*** Preserves proper alkalinity of body fluids Absorbed from the small intestine Deficiencies caused by hormone products	B complex D Calcium

(Minerals)

Mineral	Sources	Assists / maintains	Synergises with
Selenium	*Liver, kidney*	An antioxidant	B₃
	Crab, oysters, tuna, mackerel, herrings	Glutathione metabolism	C
	AFA, spirulina	Protection of cell membranes	E
	Mushrooms, cucumber, broccoli, cabbage, asparagus, radish, onions, garlic, alfalfa sprouts	Detoxification from chemicals	Iron
	Brazil nuts, cashews, *peanuts*		Zinc
	Wholegrain cereals	*Noteworthy*	Methionine
	Brewer's and torula yeast, molasses	Stimulates the immune system	Cysteine
	Eggs, *chicken, chicken liver*	Inhibits lipid peroxidation	Co-enzyme Q₁₀
		Necessary for a healthy male reproduction system; promotes normal body growth and fertility in both sexes	
		Necessary for the production of prostaglandins—promotes a healthy heart	
		Absorbed in the duodenum	
		Lost through milling and refining, food processing, heating and cooking	

(Minerals)

Mineral	Sources	Assists / maintains	Synergises with
Silicon	AFA Oats, wholegrain cereals, barley Root vegetables (esp. beets/beetroot), green leafy vegetables, *peppers* Grapefruit Horsetail (equisetum) Seafood Brown rice, soybeans	Health and integrity of skin, nails, hair and blood vessels Collagen formation Decrease of cholesterol permeation into arterial walls Healthy connective tissues *Noteworthy* An antioxidant, particularly against aluminium Essential during growth periods and for bone calcification Present in skin, nail, bone and tracheal tissues, and in the lymph nodes, tendons, aorta and lungs	Boron Calcium Magnesium Manganese Potassium

(Minerals)

Mineral	Sources	Assists / maintains	Synergises with
Sodium	Tuna, clams, *crab, shrimps,* sardines, kelp *Brains, liver, ham, poultry* Celery, cabbage, watercress, beets, sauerkraut, peas Olives *Cheese, cottage cheese* *Pickles* Salt Red kidney beans Miso, soy sauce AFA, spirulina *MSG*	Digestion (necessary for the production of hydrochloric acid in the stomach) Permeability of cells Blood pressure Lymph and blood health Glucose absorption Acid base balance (in its synergistic relationship with potassium) Homeostasis of digestive and nervous systems ***Noteworthy*** Prevents dehydration; maintains the water body balance An essential mineral which is found in every body cell, especially in extra-cellular fluids (intestinal and vascular fluids) Absorbed in the small intestine and stomach	B_6 D Calcium Magnesium Phosphate Potassium

(Minerals)

Mineral	Sources	Assists / maintains	Synergises with
Sulphur	Fish Eggs *Meats* Onions, garlic, leeks, shallots, chives, cress, brussels sprouts, horseradish, spinach, cabbage, asparagus, celery, lettuce, avocado, radish, *aubergine*, dandelion, jerusalem artichokes, *potatoes*, sweet corn Pineapple, grapefruit, figs, strawberries, cherries, raisins	The formation of amino acids in the metabolism of proteins Collagen formation Bile secretion in the liver ***Noteworthy*** Prevalent in keratin A cleanser and antiseptic Topical applications used to treat psoriasis, eczema and dermatitis Absorbs water in the intestines and promotes a laxative reaction	Cysteine Methionine Taurine

(Minerals)

Mineral	Sources	Assists / maintains	Synergises with
Zinc	Beef, organ meats Turkey Oysters, herrings, crab Sunflower, pumpkin, squash seeds Milk, live yoghurt Eggs Ginger Brewer's yeast Wheat germ, brown rice, whole grains Rye bread Soybeans Mushrooms	Metabolism, through its involvement in over 80 enzyme systems Immune system functions Sensory functions Wound healing RNA and DNA synthesis Sexual and brain development Prostate function Bone and teeth formation Healthy skin and hair **Noteworthy** Synergistic with growth hormone and insulin Absorbed through the duodenum, jejunum and ileum Absorption prejudiced by excessive calcium intake (zinc, cadmium, silver and copper compete for the same absorption sites in the small intestine)	A B6 D E Magnesium Manganese Cysteine Insulin

Table 8: Acid-forming and alkaline-forming foods

Approximately 80 per cent of our diet should be comprised of alkaline-forming foods, with the remainder acid-forming foods. This conclusion is based on the results of the metabolic process, which produces leftovers, a residue which, depending on its chemical composition, can influence the blood acid/alkaline balance.

Therefore it is helpful to know what is an acid-forming food. This should not be confused, however, with the food's acidity. For example, citrus fruits are high in citric acid. This acid is fully metabolised in the digestive process; the result is actually alkaline-forming.

Use the following table to assist with planning a dietary program that leans in favour of alkaline-forming practices.

Sources which can be regarded as possible 'triggers' for psoriatics are *italicised*.

ACID		NEUTRAL	ALKALINE	
High	**Medium**		**Medium**	**High**
Meats				
Bacon	Mackerel			
Beef	Herrings			
Chicken				
Liver				
Lamb				
Veal				
Shellfish				
Fish				
Dairy Products				
Edam cheese	*Cheddar*	*Butter*	Milk (*cow*, soy, sheep, goat)	
Mayonnaise	*Stilton*	*Margarine*		
Heated milk		*Cream cheese*		

ACID		NEUTRAL	ALKALINE	
High	**Medium**		**Medium**	**High**
Nuts				
	Walnuts	Pumpkin seeds	Almonds	
	Pasta			
	Noodles			
	Corn starch			
Fruits				
	Cranberries		Citrus	Dried Fruits
	Plums		Apples	Rhubarb
	Prunes		Apricots	
	Olives		Peaches	
			Pears	
			Grapes	
			Cherries	
			Raspberries	
			Figs	
			Melons	
Vegetables				
Mustard	Butter beans	Avocado	Root vegetables	Beetroot
Cooked tomatoes and processed tomato products	Broad beans		Celery	
	Cress		Lettuce	Carrots
	Asparagus		Cabbage	*Potatoes*
	Brussels sprouts		*Tomatoes*	
	Spinach		Beans	Cress

ACID		NEUTRAL	ALKALINE	
High	**Medium**		**Medium**	**High**
Vegetables				
			Mushrooms	
			Onions	
			Corn	
				Sea vegetables
				Kelp
				Freshwater and seawater algae
Others				
Eggs		Maple syrup	Pulses	
Sugar and all products made from sugar and sweeteners		Soybeans and soy products	Molasses	
		Olives	Honey	
		Coconut	Sugar-free jams	
			Pure fruit concentrates	
			Vanilla essence/ pods	
Beverages				
Alcohol	*Coffee*	Water		All fruit juices
Tomato juice (tinned/ vacuum-packed)	*Tea*	Herb teas		Yeast extract drinks

ACID		NEUTRAL	ALKALINE	
High	**Medium**		**Medium**	**High**
Beverages				
Chocolate	Cereal and non-cereal coffee substitutes			All vegetable drinks, *tomato juice (fresh)*
	Cocoa			*Lassis*
				Fruit teas
				Dandelion coffee
Dried foods				
	Legumes	Lentils	Currants	
	Beans		Raisins	
	Chickpeas		Sultanas	
Condiments				
Ketchup, tomato sauce			Umeboshi plum	
Mustard			Miso	
Pickles			Tamari	
			Shoyu	

Table 9: Food combining—the food groups

Food	Protein	Fat	Carbohydrate	Sugar
Grains, pulses	High	Low-medium	Low-medium	
Fish, *meat*	High	Medium-high	Low-medium	
Nuts, seeds	Medium	Medium-high	Medium-high	
Eggs	Medium	Medium		
Dairy products	Low	Medium-high		
Vegetables	Very low	Low	Low-medium	
Fruit	Nil	Nil	Nil	High

Table 10: Food combining—practical applications

Sources which can be regarded as possible 'triggers' for psoriatics are *italicised*.

Food	Combines with	Should not combine with
Vegetables		
Root vegetables	Protein	Fast-fermenting fruits
Salad vegetables	Starches	
Legumes	Fruits (except fast-fermenting)	
Avocados		
Tomatoes		
Pumpkin		
Capsicum (peppers)		
Protein foods		
Meat	Vegetables	Fruits and fast-fermenting fruits
Fish		Starches

Food	Combines with	Should not combine with
Protein foods		
Poultry		
Eggs		
Cheese		
Yoghurt		
Milk		
Starches		
Potatoes	Vegetables	Protein
Bread		Fruits
Pasta		Fast-fermenting fruits
Rice		
Rye		
Oats		
Fruits		
Apples	Starches	Protein
Coconut		Fast-fermenting fruits
Bananas		
Fast-fermenting fruits		
Mango		Protein
Melon		Starches
Berries		Vegetables
Papaya (pawpaw)		Other fruits
Pears		

Table 11: Antioxidant food sources

Sources which can be regarded as possible 'triggers' for psoriatics are *italicised*.

Ascorbic acid	Carotenoids	Citric acid	Bioflavenoids	Phenolic compounds	Selenium	Tocopherols	Blood purifiers
Foods high in vitamin C (*See also* Table 6)	Yellow and orange fruit and vegetables	Citrus fruit	Green growing shoots of all plants Citrus fruits (particularly white flesh) *Red wine* Vegetable and fruit skins (*See also* Table 6)	Ginger Onions Oats Red wine Grapes Citrus fruits Vegetables Vanilla bean Sesame seeds Cereal grains Soybeans *Tea* Turmeric *Mustard*	Green and brown lentils Seeds and nuts Seafood *Meats* Cereal grains (*See also* Table 7)	*Animal protein (including vitamin E)* Carrots (excluding vitamin E activity) Cereal grains Legumes Lentils Nuts Seed oils	Asparagus Broad beans Chick peas Ginseng Kidney beans Lentils Mung beans Oats *Peanuts* Red clover Sarsaparilla Soybeans Spinach

Appendix 2:
Information exchange

With the publication of *Sor-i-a-sis* in November 1981, there evolved an information exchange to which many people contributed their own (self-healed and case history) experiences.

The following are extracts from a selection of this correspondence, together with a few updates which were provided twenty years later.

Readers' experiences

Before I received your publication I had started on the Psorin treatment ... along with your dietary information [this] has kept me completely free for six months.

Twelve years ago I had an emotional trauma which I believed triggered this psoriasis to begin with. Over the years I have believed it could be helped by food types so I tried to keep to the unrefined, additive-free as much as possible (as much as skin specialists scoffed that it was nothing to do with food—it was incurable, hereditary, you just have to live with it, etc., etc.).

Your book supported (though vastly improved on) my theories with regards food. Your example of successful self cure has been very encouraging to me and I'm sure to every fellow sufferer who reads it.

Miss R.S., Brisbane

The skin disease I had for years has all cleared up. I have been eating raw foods also made up an ointment of the plant Hyssop. It's the famous Biblical plant (see *Psalms* 51: 7). Also I did take some of the plant in my food every 4 days, it worked so fast. Also for four years I had haemorrhoids so bad I did try all kinds of things. No good, but Hyssop was the cure for that and psoriasis. I thank you for telling me to eat the right food.

C. G. R., DHM, Western Australia

C.G.R., who trained in herbal medicine, provided directions for making hyssop tea and the hyssop ointment, as follows:

Hyssop (*Hyssopus officialis*) is an old herb once widely cultivated for medicinal use. It is now grown mostly as an ornamental shrub.

Properties and uses Astringent, carminative, emmenagogue, expectorant, stimulant, stomachic, tonic.

Hyssop tea Steep 1 tsp of dried leaves in ½ cup of boiling water. Sweeten with honey. Take every 4 days.

Hyssop ointment Take 1 cup of fresh hyssop leaves. Bruise them and beat together with hard honey. Place in a glass jar in the sun for one week and then freeze until set.

C.G.R. stipulates hard honey. It also figures in this remedy against viruses:

Take 2 tsps of thyme. Boil in 1 cup of water. When ready to drink, add 5 drops of eucalyptus oil and some honey. Take every 3 hours.

The best treatment I ever had was from a herbalist, but he died without passing on the secret of his remedy.

When psoriasis is an inherited condition, and there is a long history of it on my mother's side of the family, one has a lifelong struggle to cope with it, and I feel that we must have some severe chemical deficiency. In this month's *Here's Health* magazine [October 1982] I read with interest that a New Zealand engineer who noticed that animals grazing pasture rich in cobalt, iodine and potassium were free from arthritis and skin disease, developed a product called Tracel, and that human volunteers have claimed some success with it. I wonder if you have heard of that?

Miss A., Coventry, England

(This product was not available in January 2001.)

I have had the psoriasis for a number of years, when my father got ill and later passed away and [I had] a lot of personal worries. I have had it ever since, a trip to hospital helped once but it came back. I am now keeping the ailment 'at bay' by watching my diet and taking Zinvit tablets.

Mrs R., Wyong, NSW

The thought that there may be a chance of healing has brightened me very much.

I do follow a fairly healthy diet and a long while before I read your first booklet I was following Paavo Airola's course of vitamins in the large doses it specified. My psoriasis improved quite a lot but I was still dissatisfied and looking for quicker and better results—a cure.

Sun, salt water and relaxation have been highly beneficial. I have decided I would like to seek the help of a hypnotherapist. I think Step 1 in my case is to become positive of a cure.

A.H., Warrnambool, Vic

Update 2001 On the third-last day of 2000, A.H. related via telephone how she had returned to a cold, dry climate a year earlier, following three years in a hot, sunny climate where she enjoyed clear skin. Having suffered from psoriasis since she was six years old, and been through the mill with coal tar and steroid preparations, and eventually having established a sound understanding of natural health, A. described her annoyance at the re-emergence of the familiar spots within the past year.

Psoriasis has shown hereditary links in A.'s family, with her sister breaking out pre-nuptials, and with complete remission following her marriage; mother and a brother occasionally have the symptoms.

When asked whether or not she had pursued hypnotherapy, A. replied that she had never found 'the right person' in whom to place her faith.

A. believes in the importance of cleansing and has undertaken a Cabot liver-cleansing program. She is currently using Psori Lotion, containing chamomile, chickweed and nettle extracts, and lime and tea-tree oils, which she describes as beneficial.

My body is being taken over by psoriasis. I've had it for seventeen years now and it has disappeared during this time. But now it is developing in my fingernails and my scalp is a mass of it. I can't understand why. I follow a relatively healthy diet. Plenty of fresh fruit and vegies.

Further correspondence several months later revealed:

... the psoriasis on my nails—fingers—with the continual application of Lucas' Pawpaw Ointment has gone into remission and the new nail is healthy and strong. Also I have seen good results with Jojoba Creme— Nature's Own Magic by Bergel, California.

Rosemary oil and non-chemical shampoos and conditioners have helped considerably.

Mine stems from a physical reaction as a result of insupportable stress and pressure in my life. I also feel that it may be a particular trace element I am missing or that I'm not eating or assimilating enough protein. I am allergic to dairy products and prefer non-mucous-forming foodstuffs.

Ms M., Liverpool, NSW

I am 31 years old and have suffered with psoriasis for 28 years. Although I believe [it] is only the result of body organs not functioning to their capacity, I firmly believe there is a way of increasing their functions to maintain a good body balance and rid the skin affliction.

I turned vegetarian 5½ years ago and my skin has been slowly improving to a point where I am not getting any better or any worse.

We grow most of our own food and it is organic. It appears to me that herbs (e.g. dandelion leaf tea, alfalfa, etc.), good diet, a neutral pH body level and positive state of mind all help to rid this affliction.

Mrs S., Cowaramup, WA

Update 2001 I have suffered for 46 years. I believe this affliction is only the result of body organs not functioning to their capacity. My philosophy is to maintain a level of health of mind and body, before reducing or totally eliminating ... this affliction. Overall health has been and still is improving after turning vegetarian 24 years ago. The line of thought, 'We may have been born with a weakness [psoriasis] but it does not mean we have to always have it', is constantly in my mind. I firmly believe that the only way to rid this affliction is time, patience and the correct recipe for each individual. The more natural, the better. Psoriasis is only a symptom, not a disease. My improvement would be rated at 90 per cent since first starting on a self-help program.

Mrs S.'s mother first developed signs of psoriasis at age 75 (in 2000). Her daughter has it very mildly.

She cites the power of the mind as being very important and effective. Mrs S. had achieved 'astonishing results' after six weeks of maintaining a practice of looking at her skin and telling the psoriasis to 'go, go, go'. This state was maintained until Mrs S. was acutely poisoned by an organophosphate spray in the mid-1990s. She states that if it were not for this and the death of her father about three years later, her psoriasis would not be with her today.

Mrs S. is adamant that diet and mind power are more effective than surface treatments, and that natural therapies are more appropriate than medical intervention. The 'number one step' for Mrs S. was changing from a heavy red meat diet 25 years ago, and today she is driven by the positive attitude that she will 'not leave this earth with the symptom of the weakness'.

I have it on my elbows where it is just begging to heal and have it on penis (apparently healed) and scrotum (nearly healed).

P.F., Ainslie, ACT

Four months later:

My skin has not improved, and I realise that I must do more if I want to be rid of it. I have some habits which probably aren't helping and I find them difficult to throw away.

Over the last couple of years I have reverted to some old habits— drinking coffee, beer, wine, smoking. In doing so I realise I am merely re-intoxicating my body, with the net result of another toxaemic condition unless I regularly detoxify. Ultimately, our health is in our own hands, no doubt a platitude to you, but rather than get hung up on that, it is necessary if we are to be healthy and happy to strike a balance between what we need and what is required of us in the world at large.

A further two months later:

There has been some improvement since I last wrote. It's a little hard to isolate what has been responsible—around about the same time the following happened—I gave away smoking, drinking coffee and alcohol, started yoga, practised a relaxation technique, [and] started using calendula cream and bergamot oil.

I am a sufferer of psoriasis, have been for 3 years. I'm 48 years old, a bit overweight, and I have four daughters. My main area is my scalp, some on my elbows and knees. I get so ashamed every time I go to have my hair cut. Can't have a perm.

Ms D., Tamworth, NSW

I too have had it; and all specialists said no cure—so I have cured myself hopefully, as I have been clear of it for 12 months.

Mrs T., Inverell, NSW

Mrs T. briefly described her regimen as follows:

No soap in the bath at all, instead Alpha Keri oil added to the bath water.

A multi-vitamin formula, 1 tablet at each meal and reducing this to 1 tablet per day as improvement showed.

100IU of vitamin E at each meal, and reducing to 1 per day.

Alpha Keri oil (a tar-based product) is still available.

I have the complaint very badly. Mine is the type which is much worse in the summer. I am covered with it though my body is a lot better this year. I have resorted to homeopathic medicine after 48 years under doctors, specialists, etc. I have had homeopathic treatment for nearly three years and am a lot better, but have a long way to go.

Mrs G., Derbyshire, England

Three months later:

My Homeopathic Doctor said that you were thinking on the right lines and positive thought such as yours is a great help. I am gradually changing my diet but not too quickly, as my doctor thinks that one should not be too drastic as the body has to have time to adjust. I am clearing up much earlier. I did try to get the Bloodwood but our Herbalists are not allowed to sell it any more.

I have suffered from psoriasis for the past four years and have found the only thing so far which will remove the rash is sunbathing for short times each day, but would like something for winter treatment.

L.B., Tasmania

I have known for many years about diet etc., having been a vegetarian since 1940, and believe that Naturopaths and Herbalists are the real Doctors. I wouldn't go along with Acupuncture or Hypnotherapy, also Reincarnation is not accepted by any person who claims to be a Christian.

Mr C., Sussex, England

On reincarnation In the 6th century AD, the Emperor Justinian, who was even more corrupt than Constantine, came up against the difficulty that even soldiers who had obtained 'absolution' were afraid of the karmic possibilities of reincarnation and rebirth. He therefore set about the final abolition of belief in reincarnation, hitherto a part of Christian teaching. (Source: Dennis Stoll, 'New Light From Ancient Egypt', in *COSMOS The Living Paper*, Vol. 10 No. 1, August 1982.)

My request for the book was actually to discover how to correct psoriasis on my 14-month-old son. Your book has certainly assisted as far as the external [surface] healing suggestions [are concerned] and certainly many of the dietary changes could be useful. In many cases it is difficult to adapt them to the palate (and lack of teeth!) of a baby, however.

If my son's ailment has been accurately diagnosed [since confirmed] then I wonder if this would 'soften' your view of the importance of one's mental attitude re the 'within'. Unless teething could be considered as stress, I would not see emotions as playing a great part in this instance.

Further correspondence raised these points:

By palate I really meant that if a child doesn't like something, e.g. raw tomato, some fruits etc., or the taste of bean soup, there is not much that can be done about it. Currently I am trying to offer as many different raw fruits and vegetables as possible but with little success. I've ended up sneaking them into favoured foods where possible.

I would most certainly agree that teething causes stress. However, it is a physical stress rather than an emotional one. In my son's case it appears that whenever his body goes into an imbalance, the psoriasis reappears. So far possible causes of imbalance have been fluoride drops, measles vaccination, and gastric attack, as well as less obvious dietary 'mishaps'.

PS Apricot kernel oil in the bath is good.

Mrs D., Vic

Update 2001 Mrs D.'s son has escaped psoriasis. He is nineteen years old at the time of writing, and apart from flare-ups when he was particularly stressed, when some spots did appear including on his face, the lad gained a long-term remission. Mrs D. described her son's skin as always being very sensitive, and in teenage years he experienced severe acne which passed in time. Her father had very sensitive skin and her brother experenced 'amazing skin reactions'.

A further development in March 2001 caused Mrs D. to relate news of a recent diagnosis of pompholyx (cheiropompholyx) in the arch of her foot.

This is an itchy eczematous condition which is sometimes mistaken for psoriasis, arises in those who are given to profuse sweating, and is difficult to treat. Mrs D.'s doctor prescribed cortisone, which she has not used, instead opting for natural 'wild weed ointment', bergamot oil and pawpaw cream.

I have just read your article, and I think the only person to talk to about Psoriasis is an experienced person.

I am 16 and first got psoriasis a few years ago but it only lasted a couple of months, but just last year it came back and I have had it now for about 6 months.

Having visited a number of doctors I have just about given up, because half of them tell me what it is (as if I don't know already) but don't give me anything for it.

I think it could be emotional. It doesn't bug me that much but I don't fancy wearing bikinis all the time, it gets a bit embarrassing. The worst place I have it is all over my stomach, my elbows, knees, on my arms and legs, and back in a few places.

So I am interested in reading your book. I haven't done anything much about it, so I thought I'd better get rid of it.

My boyfriend isn't too keen on them either, he always calls me a leopard.

J.S., Kingscliff, NSW

I am J.'s mother. I found the letter she had written to you in her drawer (weeks after) so I posted it to you. When she said she was writing, I said, he will tell you similar to what I have told you (starting with diet). Hence, I guess this is why she didn't follow through—they (adolescents) do not want to be different to their friends at 16.

I am a yoga teacher. We eat all of the foods you mention. J. and her boyfriend prefer to go out and live on takeaways. If we were on polluted foods she would probably be a 'Health Crank'. I am hoping that reading your words, an outsider who has had it, will make her stop and take a step in the right direction.

Later correspondence:

The surface healing is all J. wishes to do at the moment. She is eating out everywhere but at home. The zinc sits in the cupboard with all the other vitamins and minerals.

Four months later:

J. is still having more milk than is best for her, but at least I have managed to have her here for more meals—lovely, just cooked vegies in stainless steel. She is also exercising two classes a week, so it is a breakthrough, she never touches tea or coffee, only herbal. She will come around eventually, they see how well you are.

She is a 2nd year hairdressing apprentice. The whole thing is with the chemicals and hairsprays, her skin was ok before she started her career, so that's another thought.

E.S., Kingscliff, NSW

When I was pregnant with my second child, psoriasis appeared out of nowhere. It started on my elbows, and my legs were covered in the scales. When the child was born, a boy, the psoriasis left my legs as quickly as it had come. After my third child, also a boy, psoriasis again appeared on my legs for about six to nine months and then again left. I had no more children and no more psoriasis of the legs. It did remain on my elbows and is still there.

One week after originally getting psoriasis, my sister, who is five years older, also developed it. She thought she had caught it from me, but the doctor assured her this was not so as it's not catching, but we both felt it was odd that she got it a week after I did—as children she was the sister who caught everything I had. My oldest sister, who was in closer contact with me, never caught my mumps or measles or whatever, although she did have various other illnesses as a child. My brother, mother and oldest sister all had eczema, my other sister and myself having psoriasis. She has completely ridden herself of it now, hers was through her scalp, around her ears, small patch on her face. I don't think she had it on her body much. My first child was a girl (no incidence of psoriasis).

Mrs B., Berowra Heights, NSW

I am delighted with your book, I will start its application soon. I know you are right on to the cure, as you say, minor adjustments and success. Thank you for all you have done for all of us, I know how you have suffered being an ex-sufferer myself—I actually used a very similar method. Thank you a thousand times.

Naturopath, Sydney, NSW

I am writing on behalf of my mother who is 80 years old and has been a psoriasis sufferer for many, many years. She has been attending doctors who keep assuring her that there really is no cure for the disease and soothing ointment is the only treatment. My mother accepts the 'inevitability' of the situation, but I think that if there is any chance of your treatment helping her avoid her daily sufferings, then it should be tried; very expensive treatments are out of the question.

Mrs P.C., Seaford, Vic

Five months later:

The good medical men who were treating my mother could not be accused of not trying because they did try, but were not very successful. One of them prescribed an appointment with a specialist and when that specialist failed, went to some considerable effort to locate another man who produced an ointment which was apparently soothing and did give the lady some relief.

Mum read your booklet and relegated it to the 'too hard' bin. She said, 'I'm too old now to try changing my diet and habits. It wouldn't be possible for me to do it.' However, only last week she decided to study the booklet again and has been asking questions on diet items, so perhaps there may be some hope of her attempting the measures recommended.

I have had this condition in my scalp for over twenty years and have searched constantly for a cure, though given little chance of succeeding by those whom I had consulted. Now, with treatment prescribed by a local specialist I think I just about have it beaten.

Mrs O., Tamworth, NSW

In response to a request for more details of her successful treatment Mrs O. provided information describing treatment beginning with Methotroxate in very small, very carefully controlled doses (following pathology tests to determine the ability of her blood, liver and kidneys to cope with the drug), Alphosyl HC lotion, changing to Diprosone cream, and finally Betnovate ½ Gel. She describes the results, a year later, as 'tremendous', and finds a personal advantage in using shampoos with a jojoba base.

I've had psoriasis for 20 years. I've tried just about every cream and vitamin pill there is, salt water and sun, yoga, meditation, breathing techniques, massaging—you name it I've tried it. I'm a vegetarian.

Helen, Sydney, NSW

Some months later:

I've also tried zinc tablets which did not help. Now I have some very interesting information for you. I [saw a] doctor [who] told me [of] some creams and tablets from Russia, but I had to get a permit from the government, which I'm still hassling with. Anyway, I got the tablets—Calgam B15—and have cured it up in two weeks. Calgam B15 is pure pangamic acid (calcium pangamate). [It] eliminates intoxications of various kinds, and influences the condition of the central nervous system. The Russian Academy of Sciences has found that psoriasis is a virus in the blood and have had great success in using B15. By the way, there is a man in Queensland who is putting out a tablet B15 which is not pure Calcium Pangamate. It's on the poisons list, so be careful. The Russians are about 20 years ahead of us and America in their research in diseases.

In two days of taking the tablets I slept better, felt a lot calmer, no butterflies in my tummy; my hot flushes disappeared, and the muck that came out of my skin was unbelievable, [with me] ending up having two showers a day (with soap) and scrubbing my skin all over with a brush. I didn't put any creams on, and another thing, it didn't itch even when I put soap on it (Sunlight brand). By the way, I stayed on a normal diet, was eating two eggs a day, fish and salad, Vogel bread and butter.

You can buy the Russian B15 overseas in most countries, in India you can pick up a bottle of 200 tablets for 50c. I've now been hassling with the Government here for two months, trying to get the permit to import the tablets. It's also legal to bring in 20,000 tablets from another country.

After providing the National Health and Medical Research Council in Canberra with an undertaking that she would not take any action against the doctor who prescribed the Calgam and two other Russian synthetic agents, Psoriasin and Oxolin, Helen finally succeeded in gaining permission to import the B15.

Some months later:

I have been doing research into Calcium Pangamate B15 and how it helps psoriasis sufferers. The liver is not functioning right. The liver is the largest organ in the body, and thousands of chemical reactions take place in it every second during life. The liver produces cholesterol, lecithin, bile, blood albumin vital to the removal of tissue wastes, prothrombin essential to the clotting of blood, and innumerable enzymes and co-enzymes. It stores iron, copper, several trace minerals, vitamin A and to some extent D, E, K and the B vitamins. A healthy liver destroys harmful substances such as poisons, chemicals and toxins from bacterial infections.

Now, what B15 does is help the liver produce its own lecithin. By doing that it starts functioning properly, and in turn a lot of things start happening in the body: all the organs that are thrown out [by the liver's malfunctioning] start functioning like they are meant to. The cholesterol level in the blood drops, improves lipid metabolism and normalises accumulated uric acid. B15 normalises the potassium and sodium levels. All of this starts happening when the liver is functioning properly, the blood is filtered of its impurities. So when the blood is clean, the oxygen in the blood assists the reproduction of the skin tissue.

I have very little to no itching any more.

Please accept my very grateful thanks for your book on Psoriasis. However, apart from one or two small points it does not tell me anything I don't already know, or haven't tried—but before you get too upset, please allow me to explain.

I am 60 years of age, and have lived with a skin condition of one sort or another for most of my life, and from my conception have had weak veins and bad circulation in the legs below the knee, which in turn has caused a bad varicose vein condition where the psoriasis now is.

My mother was of Jewish stock, my father Scottish, so many and varied was the food I ate as a child, and having a family of seven, my parents, especially during the depression of the 30s, used every sort of food they could lay their hands on, not all of it good, just filling. But that was just lack of understanding and I don't hold that against them. On the other hand, while not understanding diet, they put me to every sort of vigorous exercising and sport you could name, to strengthen my legs, and it probably did me much good. I am an extremely fit person (from the knees up, to quote my doctor), and keep as active as I possibly can.

After I was married (early 40s), pregnancy caused me many problems with leg ulcers, one which took eighteen months to close, and phlebitis, also there was always the inevitable rashes. Having exhausted all the doctors could do for me I began to look at 'natural' means of healing and right diet which improved my health considerably.

Phlebitis kept my life literally 'hanging by a thread' many times. About 4–5 years ago I had the two worst clots I had ever experienced, but a Naturopath brought them both out through the skin with Epsom salts packs on the clots and raw onion packs on the soles of the feet. I have had very little of that problem since then.

My old family doctor did every test he could for the rashes, even sending me to skin specialists. It was discovered that I have the finest of fine skins which is 'allergic to everything' to quote one of them. I had four different rashes on my body at one time, and still have two today. I was attending the Vedral Herbal Health Clinic (VHHC) at Southport (Qld). They are 'natural' skin specialists and said I had 'blood in the skin' (not infected) underneath the psoriasis. However, with right diet and ointments they were able to relieve the condition quite a lot, but as I am a pensioner and the treatment very expensive I can't keep it up.

The main thing I would like improved is the itch and this poses a problem. Because of the irreparable damage that clots and ulcers have done to my legs in the past, I have to keep them bandaged to force the blood down to the feet and up again, and this does nothing for the itch. But I try all that is suggested to me and I thank God that He has granted me the measure of health I have at my age. I have deep religious belief, and study the Bible on God's Laws of food, fasting, cleanliness, sunshine, fresh air, exercise, sleep, rest, diet and elimination, bodily injury, and above all keeping a positive mental attitude.

My life was not easy in the past and probably emotional upsets did not help any, but I have learned to overcome them, and have a strong loving family behind me. I have all the books on natural healing for my particular problem and feel I have gone as far as I can go. I worked out a diet that suits me from VHHC's chart and Paavo Airola's list of vitamins, including zinc, seem to suit me best. I also have 3–4 of the oils you mention. Unfortunately we only have chlorinated water (we are not allowed tanks up here) and the sea water in Moreton Bay is extremely dirty. I do put Epsom salts or apple cider vinegar in the bath water to help. I have got an assortment of ointments etc., but because of the condition under the psoriasis many of them are too strong. If they are mild enough to use, they only help for a short while, then the condition reverts back to what it was.

I will keep trying, but I know the ultimate healer is God. He told the ancient Israelites (of whom we are all descendants) that if they obeyed His Laws, Commandments and Statutes, He would put 'none of these diseases' on them (Exodus 15:26), and that is still true today. We bring these curses upon ourselves, for if we break a law, it will exact a penalty, and more times than enough in illness.

We could lessen all our problems if we would just stop and think how we live, what we eat, even how we think, etc. I know it has made a marvellous difference to my life since I have tried to practise this.

Mrs B., Brisbane, Qld

Two months later:

I have been given a new treatment to see if it worked, and the results have been astounding. Apply twice a day equal parts of Wheatgerm oil and Claret (mixed). Either rub well into the condition, or soak bandage in mixture and apply firmly (depending on where condition is). This has almost faded out the 'red area' under the psoriasis, and the scale has almost gone, the itch has gone completely.

I have not had so much comfort in years. I thought I would pass it on for what it's worth. Someone else may be helped by it. All the best.

Contact with other psoriatics also resulted from a magazine article published in 1984. This reader ventured the following information in December 2000.

I really feel ... the bad times are almost always in stressful times. About seven years ago I [was] under a specialist [and was] introduced to the PUVA treatment which was great to break the cycle and return the skin to normal.

I eat quite a balanced diet and I don't drink any alcohol at all. If I was to drink red wine my skin would itch and erupt immediately.

At this time I am managing quite well with just a few spots. My weight has increased over the years. Over the last three months I have attend[ed] the gym [and] really feel great for this. I have consciously made the decision to go to the gym even if the skin is not clear, I just [cover up with] a tracksuit. I've used psoriasis as an excuse in the past. I feel I have broken through this barrier.

I try to drink 10 glasses of water a day as a cleansing process.

My personal opinion is that this psoriasis is very much stress related and eating the correct diet is most important, e.g. fresh vegetables and fruits.

L.S., Melbourne, Vic.

www.psoriasis-infoexchange.com

The Information Exchange continues. In the spirit of open exchange of information and to facilitate ongoing research, submissions are invited from readers who care to share their own experiences.

If you would like to contribute information to future editions of this work, you can do so by using the facilities provided on the website— www.psoriasisinfoexchange.com.

By submitting your information you should also accept that this confers the author's permission for reprinting, and removes any obligation on the author or his publisher for compensation or payment in any form.

No names or addresses will be sought or used.

Any information submitted will be used only in future editions of this work. Privacy and security are of paramount importance—therefore absolutely no information of any kind will be provided to any third party whatsoever.

Glossary

Acetylcholine A fluid substance which transmits nerve signals.

Acidophilus bacteria (*Lactobacillus acidophilus*) Obtained from yoghurt culture, this restores the balance of intestinal bacteria.

Alkaloids A group of potent, nitrogen-containing alkaline substances.

Allopathy The orthodox treatment of illness by administering remedies which produce opposite results from the symptoms. The term was coined by Dr Samuel Hahnemann, the founder of homeopathy.

Amines Nitrogenous organic compounds.

Antioxidants Substances which counteract excess oxidation.

Arachidonic acid One of the essential fatty acids.

Astringent An agent that causes contraction of muscular fibre or vessels.

Autoimmune disease The occurrence of imbalance in the body which results from the immune system's mistaking self cells as a threat and mounting an inappropriate defence.

Azulene An oleaginous substance which imparts the herb chamomile's anti-inflammatory character.

Bioflavenoids The group name for 3,000 substances which are the main source of yellow, green and red pigments in plants. Many (notably isoflavones, such as the phytoestrogen in the soybean) have antioxidant properties.

Blood–brain barrier The cellular wall that prevents some drugs and cells from penetrating the brain.

Bromelain A digestive enzyme in fresh pineapple.

Carminative An agent for expelling gas from the intestines.

Carotenoids Naturally occurring compounds in vegetables and fruits, of which beta-carotene is one.

Chalones Control substances secreted in cells which affect the slowing or stopping of cell growth and reproduction.

Chamazulene An oleaginous substance responsible for anti-inflammatory action in the herb chamomile.

Cholinesterase An enzyme that affects nerve transmission via acetylcholine.

Cicatrise To heal over a wound, to form scar tissue.

Collagen A protein, the connective tissue which makes up 70 per cent of the skin.

Collective consciousness The grouping of all minds either in or out of harmony with each other. (Collective unconscious relates to a pool of memory, a psychic inheritance of racial experience, that is inherent in every member of the race [Carl Jung].)

Colonic irrigation The application of water introduced by an enema under pressure, together with abdominal massage, to remove old faecal matter from the bowel.

Cytokines Neurotransmitters.

Demulcent Soothing.

Ectomorph A body type characterised by long thin limbs and little fat or muscle.

Emmenagogue An agent that promotes menstrual flow.

Emollient Softening and soothing.

Endocrine glands The body's ductless glands which secrete hormones.

Endogenous Normal body inhabitants or products of our body's metabolism (e.g. friendly bacteria in the intestine; or harmful damaged or mutated cells).

Endomorph A body type intermediate between ectomorph and mesomorph.

Endorphin An opiate-like substance produced by the brain that acts as a chemical messenger to influence emotions.

Endotoxin A measurable component of certain types of bacteria.

Eosinophils Secondary white blood cells which respond to inflammatory and allergenic reactions (the state known as eosinophilia).

Epithelial cells Cells which provide a covering or lining, e.g. skin surface and intestines, blood vessels, ureter and bladder, mouth, vagina, oesophagus.

Erythema Localised redness in the skin.

Eugenics Originally the study of conditions that could improve a species, which advanced to the principle of putting to death races or individuals who do not meet a prescribed physical or mental standard.

Exanthematous Erupting skin resulting from an infectious fever.

Excitotoxin A food additive with the capability of damaging neurofunction and the immune system.

Exfoliation Peeling off the (skin's) surface.

Exogenous Materials which enter the body from the outside of the body (some are friendly, e.g. nutrients, others are hostile, e.g. viruses).

Exotoxin A toxin excreted by bacteria.

Expectorant An agent that promotes the discharge of mucus from the respiratory passages.

Extensor muscles Muscles which straighten or bend a body part.

Flavenoids Plant-derived antioxidants.

Free radicals Potentially damaging toxic substances which are created through the oxidisation of nearby molecules by unstable oxygen.

Furocoumarins Toxic chemicals which occur naturally in many foods and herbs. The synthesised furocoumarin psoralen is used in PUVA therapy.

Genes Units of heredity made up of DNA.

Glutamic acid An amino acid found in proteins.

Gluten A protein present in grains (except rice and millet).

Granulocytes White blood cells.

Haemoglobin Oxygen-carrying red blood pigment.

Halogenated salicylanides Highly photosensitive chemicals.

Histamine A substance which is produced in the bowel from the amino acid histidine. Ordinarily the enzyme histaminase, produced by the liver, makes histamine inactive.

Histidine An amino acid found in proteins.

Homeostasis Equilibrium or balance of the body state.

Homologous Naturally occurring.

Hydrogenisation A method of food processing which solidifies oils.

Hyperthyroidism Overactive thyroid gland.

Hypothyroidism Underactive thyroid gland.

Indisposition A complaint or condition.

Iridiagnosis The diagnostic principle in iridology, which examines the iris of each eye in combination with specially devised charts to determine and pre-determine health problems and therefore enable preventative therapy.

Katabolic (or catabolic) Metabolism's breaking down activity (opposite of anabolic, the constructive aspect of metabolism).

Keratin A protein found in skin and hair.

Keratinisation The process of new skin cells forming, maturing and decaying.

Keratoplastic agents Remedies for the reduction of abnormal keratinisation (also *keratolytic*).

Leaky gut syndrome A common term for the recognised condition, intestinal permeability.

Leukotrienes Intercellular messengers which are derived from essential fatty acids.

Levomenol Sesquiterpenic alcohol, the major active principle in the herb chamomile.

Lignans The components in plants which form the hard outer layer (as in seeds, nuts and whole grains), from which phytoestrogens are derived.

Lipids Fat and oils.

Lymphocytes White blood cells which produce antibodies in their function as a major player in cellular immunity.

Macrophages White blood cells whose main function is to clean up damaged or abnormal cells.

Meditation The practice of attaining a deep state of relaxation which further leads to the complete cycle of changes, chemical and energy, that takes place in the cells of the body, and which is responsible for the maintenance of growth and repair.

Melanin The pigment produced by melanoblasts in the basal cell layer of the skin which gives skin its colour.

Mesomorph A body type characterised by short strong limbs and heavy musculature.

Metabolism The conversion and utilisation of fatty acids, amino acids and sugars into energy by enzymes.

Mitosis Cell division.

Monocytes Non-granulated blood cells which follow neutrophils in the process of phagocytosis. On entering target tissue they swell to many times their original size and become macrophages.

Moxibustion Heat produced by special candles used in acupuncture treatment.

Mucopolysaccharides Long-chain sugars.

Myelin The myelin sheath is the protective cover of nerve cells (nerve endings).

Neuropeptides The brain's chemical messengers, which are also found in the skin, stomach, intestines and the heart.

Neurotoxins Substances which cause neurological damage to the brain, enabled by their penetration of the blood–brain barrier.

Neurotransmitters Hormones, biochemical messengers of the nervous system that carry nerve impulses from the brain, using cell membranes throughout the body.

Neutrophils Primary blood cells central to the cleansing of the blood supply.

NK cells Natural killer cells (of the immune system).

Oedema Swelling caused by the effusion of serum-like liquid into cells in tissue spaces or into body cavities.

Oleaginous Oily or unctuous.

Orthomolecular medicine Preventative medicine characterised by administering the correct essential nutrient at the right time.

Oxidation The process and outcome of metabolism whereby glucose (energy) is provided to cells. Free radical formation is a by-product of the natural process.

Parakeratosis Refers to imperfectly keratinised newly formed skin cells.

Pelotherapy The topical application of clay and similar preparations.

Pepsin The stomach enzyme which digests protein.

Peptides Hormones, chemical messengers which are made available through the digestion of any food containing protein and which are manufactured and stored in the brain and nerves.

Peristalsis The rhythmic contraction of the bowel which facilitates the passage of food substances during digestion.

Phagocytosis The process wherein cells such as leucocytes surround, absorb and destroy bacteria and cellular debris in the blood.

Phenol Carbolic acid, an extremely poisonous derivative of coal tar.

Phospholipids The lecithins class of fats.

Photosensitive An agent which is sensitive to sunlight.

Phytoestrogen Compounds in plants which have estrogen-like forms.

Plaque Desquamative skin, the characteristic white scale of psoriasis on the surface of the skin.

Predisposition A tendency or inclination.

Prostaglandins Hormone-like substances derived from essential fatty acids.

Proteases Amino acids.

Proteolytic Hydrolysing, or breaking down proteins into amino acids and peptides.

Prothrombin A substance in blood plasma with a direct relationship with blood clotting.

Psoralen A furocoumarin which occurs naturally in the body to make our skin sensitive to light, and in its synthetic form a key component of PUVA therapy.

Psychoneuroimmunology The study of the relationship between the mind, the nervous system and the immune system.

Purines Uric acid production is stimulated from these substances which are present in many foods.

Quercetin A polyphenol and an important carotenoid antioxidant.

Salicylic acid The old name for aspirin; also referred to as salicylates, which are common in plant foods.

Saponin A fibrous compound present in plant foods and a powerful blood purifier, immune system stimulant and antidote against the toxic effects of poisons.

Self cells The body's cells which are part of its homeostasis.

Sesquiterpenic alcohol (or levomenol) The major active principle in the herb chamomile.

Solanine The poisonous alkaloid whose presence is obvious in the green potato (can cause gastric upset and headache).

Stimulant An agent that quickens or stimulates the activity of physiological processes.

Stomachic An agent that stimulates, strengthens or tones the stomach.

Symbiosis, symbiotic relationship A union which is advantageous or necessary to both parties or factors.

Systemic Pertaining to a (body) system as a whole.

T cells T lymphocytes, immune cells produced in the thymus gland.

Tonic An agent that invigorates or strengthens organs or the entire organism.

Topical Applied to the skin.

Traditional medicine Medicine practised by indigenous people, traditional Chinese medicine, Ayurvedic medicine, herbalism; therapies which employ the principles found in these and other like forms.

Trypsin An enzyme which digests protein in the small intestine.

Urticaria An allergic reaction; also called hives.

Vasodilatation Widening of the blood vessels.

Visualisation To create a mental picture with the purpose of affecting a positive physical or material change.

Wholistic medicine A medical system which views biological conditions together with the patient's personality, lifestyle and environment.

Endnotes and references

Chapter 1

1. Hodgkin, Dr Steve, *Psoriasis*,
   http://victorvalley.com/health&law/hlaw-aug/skin.htm.
2. Živković, Danijel, MD, 'Psoriasis—A Dermatological Enigma', in *Acta Med Croatica*, 1998, Vol. 52, Issue 4–5, 199–202.
3. Ibid.
4. Ibid.
5. Bock, Kenneth, MD, and Nellie Sabin, 1997, *The Road to Immunity: how to survive and thrive in a toxic world*, Pocket Books, Simon & Schuster, New York, p. 68.

Chapter 2

1. Rose, Kenneth Jon, 1988, *The Body in Time*, John Wiley & Sons, New York, p. 9.

Chapter 3

1. Levitt, B. Blake, 1995, *Electromagnetic Fields: a consumer's guide to the issues and how to protect ourselves*, Harvest, Harcourt Brace & Company, Orlando, Florida, pp. 118–9.
2. Horne, Ross, 1983, *The New Health Revolution*, Ross Horne, Sydney, p. 47.
3. Rose, Kenneth Jon, 1988, *The Body in Time*, John Wiley & Sons, New York, p. 87.
4. Science of Life Books, 1973, *Skin Troubles: Practical remedial measures, including a special seven-day diet*, Science of Life Books, Sydney, p. 36. Meanwhile cholesterol as a nutrient is cited as being deficient in problematical skin. A West Australian pharmacist, Maurice Czarniak, BSc, BPharm, FPS, has helped psoriatics with his Healfas N.M.F.™ cream which 'addresses the localised deficiency of nutrients including cholesterol'. There are three variants of the cream, including the original, one with lavender oil and one with neem oil.

5. Rose, Kenneth Jon, op. cit.,p. 84

6. Ibid, p. 80

7. Ibid, p. 14

8. Ibid, p. 44.

9. Janowitz, Henry D., MD, 1994, *Your Gut Feelings: a complete guide to living better with intestinal problems,* Oxford University Press, New York and Oxford, p. 191.

10. McMillin, David L., MA, et al, 'Systemic aspects of psoriasis: an integrative model based on intestinal etiology', Elsevier Science Inc., in *Int Med* 1999; 2:105–13, 2000.

11. Richards, Douglas G., PhD, *Dietary and Herbal Treatment of Psoriasis,* http://community-2.webtv.net/DudleyDelaney/DietaryandHerbal/.

12. Ibid.

13. ARE Health & Rejuvenation Research Centre—The Cayce Health Database, *Overview of Psoriasis,* http://www.are-cayce.com/hrrc/database/chdata/data/prpsor3a.html. Each spinal nerve has a corresponding field in the skin called a dermatome. An entire spinal nerve can be destroyed without this being apparent in the loss of sensation to the skin.

14. Richards, Douglas G., PhD, op. cit.

15. An excess of arachidonic acid is implicated in psoriasis, due to the inflammatory nature of leukotriene B4 which is produced through the conversion of arachidonic acid.

16. McMillin, David L., op. cit.

17. Chaitow, Leon, 1991, *Thorsons Guide to Amino Acids,* Thorsons, London, p. 69.

18. Polysaccharides are complex carbohydrates composed of many different chains of glucose, such as starch and glycogen. They require longer enzyme action to be broken down and absorbed.

19. Brostoff, Dr Jonathan, and Linda Gamlin, 1989, *The Complete Guide to Food Allergy and Intolerance,* Bloomsbury, London, p. 136.

20. Reference to David Suzuki's book, *David Suzuki Talks About AIDS,* is made in *Boosting Your Immune System* by Nancy Corbett, Sally Milner Publishing, Sydney, 1991, p. 24.

21. Bock, Kenneth, MD, and Nellie Sabin, 1997, *The Road to Immunity: how to survive and thrive in a toxic world,* Pocket Books, Simon & Schuster, New York, p. 68.

22. Ibid, p. 68.

23. Holford, Patrick, 1997, *The Optimum Nutrition Bible,* Judy Piatkus

(Publishers), London, p. 120.

24. The first family refers to the biological mother and father and the child/children of that union.

25. Bittersweet nightshade (*Solanum dulcamara*); deadly nightshade (*Solanum nigrum*).

26. Blaylock, Russell L., MD, 'Excitotoxins—dangerous food additives', Part 1, in *Nexus* Vol. 7, No. 4, June–July 2000, p. 33.

27. Bell, Dr Andrew, 1989, *Creative Health: beginning the journey to wellness*, Random House New Zealand, Auckland, p. 61.

28. Holford, Patrick, 1997, op. cit, p. 135.

29. Some fresh foods contain little or none of the nutrients for which they were formerly regarded as vital sources.

30. Cribbs, Gillian, 1997, *Nature's Super Food: the blue-green algae revolution*, Newleaf, Macmillan, London, p. 31.

31. Blaylock, Russell L., op. cit, p. 41.

32. Hiestand, Denie and Shelley Hiestand, 1999, *Electrical Nutrition*, ShellDen Corp, Jersey City, New Jersey, p. 110.

33. Thornton, Mark, 'NutraSweet and the sour politics of food and drugs', in *Conscious Living*, Issue No. 53, Winter 2000, Perth, pp. 30–2.

34. Hiestand, Denie and Shelley Hiestand, op. cit. p.109.

35. Thornton, Mark, op. cit.

36. Kushi, Michio, with Edward Esko, 1991, *The Macrobiotic Approach to Cancer: toward preventing and controlling cancer with diet and lifestyle*, self published, Denver, Colorado, p.14.

37. Edwards, Sharry, MEd., 'Decloaking pathogens with low-frequency sound', in *Nexus*, Vol. 7, No. 6, October–November 2000, p. 27. In other research, Chris Bleackley and a team at the University of Alberta, Toronto, Canada, described how the protein granzyme B, which is stored in granules in the immune system's natural killer cells (NKs), assists these to penetrate infected cells. Another protein called perforin is also stored in these granules. As the name suggests, perforin is capable of punching a hole in the plasma membrane that surrounds all cells. Bleackley's team isolated another protein (mannose 6–phosphate receptor or MPR) which sits on the surface of target cells. It attaches to granzyme B and sucks it into the cell. Cells which proclaim the presence of the MPR receptor are susceptible to granzyme B and NKs, while cells which do not are NK-resistant. (Source: Valerie Depraetere, 'Lifelines: getting the enemy within', *Nature* scienceupdate, Monday 6 November 2000, http://helix.nature.com/nsu/001109/001109-3.html).

Chapter 4

1. Krishnamurti, J., 1969, *Freedom From the Known*, Harper & Row, New York.
2. Science of Life Books, 1973, *Skin Troubles: practical remedial measures, including a special seven-day diet*, Science of Life Books, Sydney, pp. 41–2.
3. Walker, Norman, and G .H. Percival, 1939, *An Introduction to Dermatology*, W. Green & Son, Edinburgh, p. 352.
4. Corbett, Nancy, 1991, *Boosting Your Immune System*, Sally Milner Publishing, Sydney, pp. 32–3.
5. Davis, Adelle, 1974, *Let's Have Healthy Children*, Unwin Books, London, p. 233.
6. Airola, Paavo, 1974, *Let's Get Well*, Health Plus Publishers, Phoenix, Arizona, pp. 145–6.

Chapter 5

1. Another word with which an extraordinary degree of licence is taken is nutritious (nutrition, et al). A complimentary sachet which dropped out of a magazine proclaims the contents as being a 'nutritious energy drink'. In fact, amongst its heavily processed ingredients is aspartame. The enthusiastic blurb on the packet proclaims, 'Because you make up [this stuff] with water and not milk, it is 99% fat free.' Are we really so contemptible and dumb?
2. Is it also possible that drug companies 'dope' the samples they provide to medical practitioners, for supply to their patients? Two products and the company involved were cited in information provided by a former pharmaceuticals sales representative who resigned from the company over this issue. Allegedly the active ingredients in these topical treatments for psoriasis were increased in the doctors' samples, so their effect was pronounced. Apparently the strategy was to excite the sufferer with a rapid improvement gained from the sample, so they became an enthusiastic consumer of less potent products.
3. Vogel, Dr H.C.A., 1995, *The Nature Doctor: a manual of traditional and complementary medicine*, Bookman Press, Melbourne, p. 180.

Chapter 6

1. Walker, Norman and G. H. Percival, 1939, *An Introduction to Dermatology*, W. Green & Son, Edinburgh, p. 246.
2. A class action suit against Miralex Health Care Inc. and Hueson Pharmaceutical Corp. was brought in the British Columbia Supreme

Court in February 2001, citing injury to claimants or their having been misled, namely sufferers of psoriasis and other skin diseases, who purchased and used Miralex cream believing it to be a 'natural' product when it contained the steroid clobetasol proprionate-17. (Source: alt.support.psoriasis,alt.support.skin-diseases.psoriasis,can.legal,us.legal,misc.legal. 9 February 2001.)

3. Lee, John R., MD, with Virginia Hopkins, 1996, *What Your Doctor May Not Tell You About Menopause: the breakthrough book on natural progesterone*, Warner Books, New York, p. 253.

4. Newnham, David, 'The dirt on dirt', in *Good Weekend*, 11 November 2000, John Fairfax Publications, Sydney, pp. 75–7.

5. Torbet, Laura (ed.), 1979, *The Helena Rubinstein Book of the Sun*, Angus & Robertson, Sydney, p. 29.

6. Photosensitive chemicals are present in a long list of consumer items and widely prescribed treatments—aniline dyes, antiseptic lotions and creams, coal tars and wood tars, deodorant soaps, hexachlorophene, medicated cosmetics and sun screens, shampoos and conditioners, and synthetic detergents. They are also present in many therapeutic drugs, including some which are used to treat acne, fungal and bacterial infections, and in barbiturates and tranquillisers, oral contraceptives and oral diabetic drugs, water pills for the control of high blood pressure, and some anti-convulsive medicines.

Chapter 7

1. Finkel, Maurice, 1975, *Good Food, Good Health: the way to live longer*, Lansdowne Press, Sydney.

2. 'Newsbytes', in *Conscious Living*, Issue No. 53, Winter 2000, Perth, p. 9.

3. From an interview on ABC Radio's 2BL heard by the author.

4. The citizens of some US states are unable to enjoy certain natural health practices including herbalism. In some states, it is illegal to provide a massage to a fellow human being without a licence.

5. Stewart, Maryon, 1998, *The Phyto Factor*, Hodder Headline, Sydney, p. 23.

6. Fallon, Sally and M.G. Enig, PhD, 'Tragedy and Hype', The Third International Soy Symposium, in *Nexus*, Vol. 7, No. 3, April–May 2000, pp. 19–24; and Sheehan, Daniel M., PhD, Director of Estrogen Base Program, Division of Genetic and Reproductive Toxicology, and Daniel R. Doerge, PhD, of the National Centre for Toxicological Research, Department of Health and Human Services of the Food and Drug

Administration, in an open letter of protest against the US Food and Drug Administration's ruling which authorises use on food labels, of health claims apropos soy protein's effectiveness in reducing the risk of coronary heart disease, dated 18 February 1999 and reproduced in *Nexus*, Vol. 7, No. 6, October–November 2000, pp. 11–13. Soybeans contain phytic acid, which has been shown to hinder the absorption of calcium, iron and zinc. However phytic acid, an important isoflavone or phytoestrogen, delivers vital antioxidant properties.

7. Stewart, Maryon, op. cit. p. 12.

8. Kirschmann, Gayla J., 1996, *Nutrition Almanac*, McGraw-Hill, Singapore, p. 369.

9. Soothill, Rayner, 1996, *The Choice Guide to Vitamins and Minerals*, Choice Books, Sydney, p. 170.

10. Some products are designed, manufactured and marketed to masquerade as 'health foods' whereas they are actually chock-a-block full of bad news.

11. Le Tissier, Jackie, 1992, *Food Combining for Vegetarians: eat for health on the Hay Diet*, Thorsons, HarperCollins, London, pp. 16–17.

12. Crook, William G., MD, 1986, *The Yeast Connection: a medical breakthrough*, Vintage Books, Random House, New York, p. 219.

13. Horne, Ross, 1992, *Health and Survival in the 21st Century*, Margaret Gee Publishing, Sydney, p. 181.

14. Dux, John, and P.J. Young, 1980, *Agent Orange: the bitter harvest*, Hodder & Stoughton, Sydney, pp. 16–19.

15. Ibid, p. 89.

16. According to Joan C. Callahan who cites as sources *Lancet* 351/9113 (May 9, 1998): 1371–75, *Rachel's Environment and Health Weekly* 598 (May 8 1998); http//www.monitor.net,Rachel, and Monsanto's rGBH information at http://www.monsanto.com, when writing in *Mother Time, women, ageing and ethics*, dairy cows' periods of lactation are artificially extended by the application of a genetically engineered bovine growth hormone (rBGH). The same cows exhibit increased levels of an insulin-like growth factor (IGF-1) that is chemically identical to the IGF-1 found in humans. IGF-1 can be passed on to humans via cow's milk. Most alarming is that IGF-1 in human blood is implicated in the risk of cancer more than any other factor which had been discovered up until 1999.

Chapter 8

1. Moir, Anne and David Jessel, 1991, *BrainSex*, Mandarin, London, p. 121.
2. Corbett, Nancy, 1991, *Boosting Your Immune System*, Sally Milner Publishing, Sydney, p. 129.
3. In a survey of 6,000 Australian workers in November 2000, more than half reported that they were in the wrong job. Accountants were the most dissatisfied (71%); even those surveyed who earned more than $100,000 per year were disgruntled. The general 'dumbing down' of society and the proliferation of fast-food joints have also resulted in a plethora of low-paid, low-skilled jobs and the escalation of discontent amongst workers in the fast-food industry and the retail sector in general. Another survey indicated that approximately two-thirds of male workers would refuse a promotion or transfer if it threatened to affect their family or intimate relationships. Sixty-eight per cent of men surveyed believe they do not spend enough time with their children.
4. A couple of hours in the garden can be more therapeutic and a sounder workout than two hours of straining and stressing in the gym.
5. From a news item on ABC-TV *World at Noon*, November 2000.
6. History is littered with the lives of individuals who have made momentous discoveries which could uplift our life experience but because of one or another vested interest, their genius is ignored or buried. Amongst a myriad innovative works (the harnessing of alternating current, being the true inventor of radio, inventing fluorescent light), Tesla demonstrated the means of providing free energy to everyone on the planet. It did not produce pollution and it never went into production. In Australia, there is a brilliant fellow who has demonstrated technology which can practically and economically supply a solid meal every day to millions of starving people regardless of their beliefs.
7. The meridians have a direct relationship with the chakras. Another word from the ancient Sanskrit (meaning 'wheel of light'), the chakras are the seven principal energy centres of the etheric body. Their balance and well-being are central to the healthy relationship of the physical body, the mind and the soul, and consequently the relationship of these with the universal light or essence. The chakras are portals or gateways via which the individual's spirit and soul are receptive to both universal and mundane energies and influences. Each also has a correspondence with a specific body region or organ, and this has

direct relevance to the chakra's own purpose and association. Aromatherapy and colour therapy work with chakras to attune them (and their host) to the universal energy, to achieve a wholistic integration of inner, outer and higher selves. As with any specialised system, the practitioner's extensive knowledge is essential.

8. Levitt, B. Blake, 1995, *Electromagnetic Fields: a consumer's guide to the issues and how to protect ourselves*, Harvest, Harcourt Brace & Company, Orlando, Florida, p. 121.

9. Edwards, Sharry, MEd, 'Decloaking pathogens with low-frequency sound', in *Nexus*, Vol. 7, No. 6, October–November 2000, pp. 27–30.

10. Distel, Kay, Sound Education (Australia), 'Sound Treatments for Good Health', in *Nexus*, Vol. 4, No. 1, December 1996–January 1997, pp. 45–47.

11. Hooper, Judith, Interview with Candace Pert, in *Omni*, February 1982, pp. 63–65; 110–112.

12. From a news item on ABC-TV *World at Noon*, November 2000.

Bibliography

Airola, Paavo, 1974, *Let's Get Well*, Health Plus Publishers, Phoenix, Arizona.

—— 1979, *Are You Confused?*, Health Plus Publishers, Phoenix, Arizona.

—— 1979, *Everywoman's Book: Dr Airola's practical guide to holistic health*, Health Plus Publishers, Phoenix, Arizona.

ARE Health & Rejuvenation Research Centre—The Cayce Health Database, *Overview of Psoriasis*, http://www.are-cayce.com/hrrc/database/chdata/data/prpsor3a.html.

Barnard, Julian, 1979, *A Guide to the Bach Flower Remedies*, Julian Barnard, Whitstable, Kent.

Beckham, Nancy, 1998, *Nature's Super Foods: top 40 medicinal foods, herbs, supplements*, Thomas C. Lothian, Melbourne.

Bell, Dr Andrew, 1989, *Creative Health: beginning the journey to wellness*, Random House New Zealand, Auckland.

Bircher-Benner Clinic Staff, 1977, *Bircher-Benner Nutrition Plan for Skin Problems*, Pyramid Publications (Harcourt Brace Jovanovich), New York.

Black's Medical Dictionary, 39th edition, 1999, Gordon Macpherson (ed.), A. & C. Black, London.

Blake, Robin, 1987, *Mind Over Medicine: can the mind kill or cure?*, Pan Books, London.

Blaylock, Russell L., MD, 'Excitotoxins: dangerous food additives', *Nexus*, Vol. 7, No. 4, June–July 2000.

—— 'Excitotoxins: dangerous food additives', *Nexus*, Vol. 7, No. 5, August–September 2000.

Bock, Kenneth, MD, and Nellie Sabin, 1997, *The Road to Immunity: how to survive and thrive in a toxic world*, Pocket Books, Simon & Schuster, New York.

Brostoff, Dr Jonathan, and Linda Gamlin, 1989, *The Complete Guide to Food Allergy and Intolerance*, Bloomsbury, London.

Brown, J.A.C., 1971, *The Stein & Day International Medical Encyclopedia*, Stein & Day, New York.

Buchman, Dian Dincin, 1973, *The Complete Herbal Guide to Natural Health and Beauty*, Doubleday, New York.

Cantassium Company, 1978, *The Original Cantassium Dietary System*, The Cantassium Company, London.

Carroll, Robert Todd, 1998, *The Hundredth Monkey Phenomenon*, from The Skeptics Dictionary, http://skepdic.com/monkey.html.

Castro, Miranda, 1995, *The Complete Homeopathy Handbook: a guide to everyday health care*, Macmillan, London.

Chaitow, Leon, 1990, *Clear Body, Clear Mind*, Penguin Books, Ringwood, Victoria.

—— 1991, *Thorsons Guide to Amino Acids*, Thorsons, London.

Chapman, J.B., MD and Edward L. Perry MD, 1976, *The Biochemic Handbook*, Formur Inc., St Louis, Mo.

Cheney, Margaret, 1981, *Tesla: Man Out of Time*, Dell Publishing, Bantam Doubleday Dell, New York.

Chopra, Deepak, 1996, *The Seven Spiritual Laws of Success: a practical guide to the fulfillment of your dreams*, Transworld, Sydney.

Cohen, J.M. and M.J., 1977, *The Penguin Dictionary of Quotations*, Penguin Books, Harmondsworth.

Collison, Dr David R., 1989, *Why Do I Feel So Awful?*, Angus & Robertson, Sydney.

Colton, Katherine, 1999, *Smart Guide to Healing Foods*, John Wiley & Sons, New York.

Corbett, Nancy, 1991, *Boosting Your Immune System* (Series: Milner Healthy Living Guide), Sally Milner Publishing, Sydney.

Cribbs, Gillian, 1997, *Nature's Super Food: the blue-green algae revolution*, Newleaf, Macmillan, London.

Crook, William G., MD, 1986, *The Yeast Connection: a medical breakthrough*, Vintage Books, Random House, New York.

Crum, Jessie, 1978, *The Art of Inner Listening*, Pyramid Publications, Wheaton, Illinois.

Davies, Jill Rosemary (Series Consultant), 2000, *Milk Thistle*, Element Books, Shaftesbury, Dorset.

Davis, Adelle, 1974, *Let's Have Healthy Children*, Unwin Books, London.

de Haas, Cherie, 1993, *Natural Skin Care*, Werribee Natural Healing Centre, Werribee, Victoria.

de Langre, Jacques, 1980, *The First Book of Dō-In*, Happiness Press, Magalia, California.

Depraetere, Valerie, 2000, 'Lifelines: Getting the enemy within', *Nature* scienceupdate, http://helix.nature.com/nsu/001109/001109-3.html.

DeRungs, Maria,1986, *Healing Tones of Music*, Casa de Maria Research Center, Virginia.

De Schepper, Luc, 1991, *Full of Life*, Tale Weaver Publishing, Los Angeles.

Distel, Kay, Sound Education (Australia), 'Sound treatments for good health', *Nexus*, Vol. 4, No. 1, December 1996–January 1997, pp.45–47.

Durant, Will, 1960, *The Story of Philosophy: the lives and opinions of the world's greatest philosophers*, The Pocket Library, New York.

Dux, John, and P.J. Young, 1980, *Agent Orange: the bitter harvest*, Hodder & Stoughton, Sydney.

Edwards, Sharry, MEd, 'Decloaking pathogens with low-frequency sound', *Nexus*, Vol. 7, No. 6, October–November 2000.

Emmerson, Ronald W., Lennart Juhlin, Terence J. Ryan, Richard A.C. Hughes and Bryan Mathews, 1980, 'Skin disorders Parts 1 and 2', *Medicine Australia Journal*, October and November 1980.

Encyclopaedia Britannica, 1962 ed. S.v. 'Anthraquinone,' by J. H. Ss.

Evans, Dr William J. and Irwin H. Rosenberg, with Jacqueline Thompson, 1992, *Biomarkers: the 10 keys to prolonging vitality*, Fireside, Simon & Schuster, New York.

Fallon, Sally and M.G. Enig, PhD, 'Tragedy and Hype', The Third International Soy Symposium, *Nexus*, Vol. 7, No. 3, April–May 2000.

Finkel, Maurice, 1975, *Good Food, Good Health: the way to live longer*, Lansdowne Press, Sydney.

Frissell, Bob, 1994, *Nothing in This Book is True, but It's Exactly How Things Are*, Frog Ltd, Berkeley, California.

Fuller, John G., 1989, *Edgar Cayce Answers Life's 10 Most Important Questions*, Warner Books, New York.

Gach, Michael Reed, 1992, *Acupressure: how to cure common ailments the natural way*, Judy Piatkus (Publishers), London.

Garten, M.O., 1967, *The Health Secrets of a Naturopathic Doctor*, Parker Publishing, West Nyack, New York.

Gibbons, Sandra, 1992, *Beat Psoriasis: simple and effective treatment—the natural way*, Thorsons, London.

Gottlieb, Karen, PhD, 1980, *Aloe Vera Heals—The Scientific Facts*, Royal Publications, Denver, Colorado.

Guyton, Arthur C., 1985, *Anatomy and Physiology*, CBS College Publishing, New York.

Haldane, J.B.S., 1937, *Possible Worlds and Other Essays*, Chatto & Windus, London.

Hall, Dorothy, 1976, *The Book of Herbs*, Pan Books, London.

—— 1976, *The Natural Health Book*, Thomas Nelson, Melbourne.

Harris, Thomas A., MD, 1973, *I'm OK—You're OK*, Cape, London.

Hay, Louise L., 1988, *You Can Heal Your Life*, Specialist Publications, Sydney.

Hiestand, Denie and Shelley Hiestand, 1999, *Electrical Nutrition*, ShellDen Corp., Jersey City, New Jersey.

Hodgkin, Dr Steve, 2000, *Psoriasis*, http://victorvalley.com/health&law/hlaw-aug/skin.htm.

Holford, Patrick, 1997, *The Optimum Nutrition Bible*, Judy Piatkus (Publishers), London.

Hooper, Judith, Interview with Candace Pert, *Omni*, February 1982, Omni Publications International Ltd., Volume 4, No. 5.

Horne, Ross, 1983, *The New Health Revolution*, Ross Horne, Sydney.

—— 1992, *Health and Survival in the 21st Century*, Margaret Gee Publishing, Sydney.

Inglis, Brian, 1964, *Fringe Medicine*, Faber & Faber, London.

Janowitz, Henry D., MD, 1994, *Your Gut Feelings: a complete guide to living better with intestinal problems*, Oxford University Press, New York and Oxford.

Jones, Dorothea Van Gundy, 1963, *The Soybean Cookbook*, Arco Publishing, New York.

Jung, Carl G. and M.-L. von Franz (eds), 1978, *Man and His Symbols*, Picador, Pan Books, London.

Kaye, Anna and Don C. Matcham, 1978, *Mirror of the Body: reflexology for good health*, Wilshire Book Company, San Francisco.

Kirschmann, Gayla J., 1996, *Nutrition Almanac*, McGraw-Hill, Singapore.

Koonin, Dr Paul M., 1941, *Health Cocktails—how to make them*, self-published, Sydney.

Krebs, Dr Charles and Jenny Brown, 1998, *A Revolutionary Way of Thinking*, Hill of Content, Melbourne.

Krishnamurti, J., 1969, *Freedom from the Known*, Harper & Row, New York.

Kushi, Michio, with Edward Esko, 1991, *The Macrobiotic Approach to Cancer: toward preventing and controlling cancer with diet and lifestyle*, self-published, Denver, Colorado.

Lee, John R., MD, with Virginia Hopkins, 1996, *What Your Doctor May Not Tell You About Menopause—The Breakthrough Book on Natural Progesterone*, Warner Books, New York.

Le Tissier, Jackie, 1992, *Food Combining for Vegetarians: eat for health on the Hay Diet*, Thorsons, HarperCollins, London.

Levitt, B. Blake, 1995, *Electromagnetic Fields: a consumer's guide to the issues and how to protect ourselves*, Harvest, Harcourt Brace & Company, Orlando, Florida.

Locke, David M., 1969, *Enzymes: the agents of life*, Crown Publishers, New York.

Longgood, William, 1969, *The Poisons in Your Food*, Pyramid Communications, New York.

Lust, John, 1974, *The Herb Book*, Bantam, New York.

McCully, Robert S., 1987, *Jung and Rorschach*, Spring Publications, Dallas, Texas.

Macfadden, Bernarr, 1937, *Encyclopaedia of Health*, Macfadden Book Company, New York.

McMillin, David L., MA, Donald G. Richards, PhD, Eric A. Meen, MD, and Carl D. Nelson, DC, 'Systemic aspects of psoriasis: an integrative model based on intestinal etiology', Elsevier Science Inc., *Int Med* 1999; 2:105–13, 2000.

Maddison, Paschale, 1999, *Healing with Clay: an introductory guide to pelotherapy*, Wildwood Sanctuary, Australia.

Miller, Sigmund Stephen, 1979, *Symptoms: The Complete Home Medical Encyclopaedia*, Pan Books in association with Macmillan, London.

Mitton, F. and V. Mitton, 1982, *Mitton's Practical Modern Herbal*, W. Foulsham & Co., Slough, Berkshire.

Moir, Anne, and David Jessel, 1991, *BrainSex*, Mandarin, London.

Newnham, David, 'The dirt on dirt', *Good Weekend*, November 11, 2000, John Fairfax Publications, Sydney.

Norris, P.E., 1960, *Everything You Want to Know About Vitamins*, Pyramid Communications Inc., New York.

Orbis Publishing, 1995, *A–Z of Natural Remedies*, Blitz Editions, Bookmart, Enderby, Leicester.

Orton, Mildred Ellen, 1978, *Cooking with Wholegrains: the basic wholegrain cookbook*, Farrar, Strauss & Giroux, New York.

Osiecki, Henry, 1990, *Nutrients in Profile*, Bioconcepts Publishing, Brisbane.

Playfair, Dr A.S., 1980, *The Hamlyn Pocket Medical Dictionary*, The Hamlyn Publishing Group, Middlesex.

Porter, Suzanne, 1988, *Understanding Cholesterol*, Suzanne Porter, Rosebud, Victoria.

Praetorius, Martin, 1972, *Nutritious Recipes and Meals*, FIT Investments, Sydney.

Reader's Digest, 1997, *Foods That Harm, Foods That Heal*, Reader's Digest, Sydney.

Restak, Richard, MD, 1991, *The Brain has a Mind of its Own*, Crown Publishers, New York.

Richards, Douglas G., PhD, *Dietary and Herbal Treatment of Psoriasis*, http://community-2.webtv.net/DudleyDelaney/DietaryandHerbal/.

Ries, Al and Jack Trout, 1986, *Positioning: The Battle for Your Mind*, McGraw-Hill, Singapore.

Rose, Kenneth Jon, 1988, *The Body In Time*, John Wiley & Sons, New York.

Ross, Janet S. and Kathleen J.W. Wilson, 1973, *Foundations of Anatomy and Physiology*, Churchill Livingstone, Edinburgh.

Russell, Bertrand, 1961, *History of Western Philosophy*, Routledge, London.

Saxelby, Catherine, 1987, *Nutrition for Life*, Reed Books, Sydney.

Science of Life Books, 1973, *Skin Troubles: practical remedial measures, including a special seven-day diet*, Science of Life Books, Sydney.

Sharon, Michael, 1989, *Complete Nutrition: how to live in total health*, Prion, Multimedia Books, London.

Sheehan, Daniel M., PhD, and Daniel R. Doerge, PhD, 'Scientists protest FDA's soy protein ruling' in deBriefings, *Nexus*, Vol. 7, No. 6, October–November 2000.

Shelton, Herbert M., 1951, *Food Combining Made Easy*, Dr Shelton's Health School, San Antonio, Texas.

Sichel, Greta, 1990, *Relief From Candida, Allergies and Ill Health*, Sally Milner Publishing, Sydney.

Soothill, Rayner, 1996, *The Choice Guide to Vitamins and Minerals*, Choice Books, Sydney.

Stanton, Rosemary and The Gut Foundation, 1994, *The Good Gut Cook Book*, Bay Books, HarperCollins, Sydney.

Stewart, Maryon, 1998, *The Phyto Factor*, Hodder Headline, Sydney.

Thornton, Mark, 'NutraSweet and the sour politics of food and drugs', *Conscious Living*, Issue No. 53, Winter 2000, Perth.

Tietze, Harald W., 1995, *Water Medicine*, Harald W. Tietze, Bermagui South, New South Wales.

Torbet, Laura (ed.), 1979, *The Helena Rubinstein Book of the Sun*, Angus & Robertson, Sydney.

Trimmer, Dr Eric, 1998, *Selenium: the trace element for health and life extension*, Thorsons, Wellingborough, Northamptonshire.

Trussell, K.W., 1981, *Sor-i-a-sis—Heal Yourself*, Cherrytree Communications, Brunswick Heads, New South Wales.

Turkington, Carol A. and Jeffrey S. Dover, MD, 1996, *Skin Deep: an A–Z of skin disorders, treatments and health*, self-published.

Vogel, Dr H.C.A., 1995, *The Nature Doctor: a manual of traditional and complementary medicine*, Bookman Press, Melbourne.

Wade, Carlson, 1972, *Nature's Cures*, Award Books, New York.

Walker, Margaret Urban (ed.), 1999, *Mother Time — women, aging and ethics*, Roman and Littlefield Publishers Inc., Maryland.

Walker, Norman, and G.H. Percival, 1939, *An Introduction to Dermatology*, W. Green & Son, Edinburgh.

Warrier, Gopi and Deepika Gunawant MD, 1997, *The Complete Illustrated Guide to Ayurveda, the Ancient Indian Healing Tradition*, Element Books, Penguin, Ringwood, Victoria.

Wilson, Colin, 1973, *The Mind Parasites*, Corgi, London.

Wilson, Colin, and John Grant (eds), 1982, *The Directory of Possibilities*, Corgi, London.

Wilson, Geoffrey D., 1988, *Food is Energy: how to use it*, Boolarong Publications, Brisbane.

Živković, Danijel, MD, 1998, 'Psoriasis—A Dermatological Enigma', in *Acta Med Croatica*, Zagreb.

Index